3 4143 10095 6232

D1578701

WITHDRAWN FOR SALE

Happy Adults

Cathy Glass

Happy Adults

WARRINGTON BOROUGH COUNCIL	
34143100956232	
Bertrams	10/02/2012
AN	£7.99
LYM	

HARPER

HARPER

An Imprint of HarperCollins*Publishers*
77–85 Fulham Palace Road,
Hammersmith, London W6 8JB

www.harpercollins.co.uk

First published by HarperCollins*Publishers* 2012

1

© Cathy Glass 2012

Cathy Glass asserts the moral right to
be identified as the author of this work

A catalogue record of this book is
available from the British Library

ISBN 978-0-00-744270-6

Printed and bound in Great Britain by
Clays Ltd, St Ives plc

All rights reserved. No part of this publication may be
reproduced, stored in a retrieval system, or transmitted,
in any form or by any means, electronic, mechanical,
photocopying, recording or otherwise, without the prior
written permission of the publishers.

MIX
Paper from
responsible sources
FSC **FSC™ C007454**
www.fsc.org

FSC™ is a non-profit international organisation established to promote
the responsible management of the world's forests. Products carrying the
FSC label are independently certified to assure consumers that they come
from forests that are managed to meet the social, economic and
ecological needs of present and future generations,
and other controlled sources.

Find out more about HarperCollins and the environment at
www.harpercollins.co.uk/green

We are only limited by the extent of our imagination
and no act of kindness, however small,
is ever wasted.

Acknowledgements

Many thanks to my editor Anne, to my agent Andrew Lownie, and to Carole, Simon and all the team at HarperCollins.

Contents

Introduction: Why?

Why do I think I have found the secret to achieving lasting happiness and contentment? Simply because I know my formula works. I have the proof.

Let me explain.

After the publication of my fostering memoirs, in which I tell the often harrowing stories of the children I've looked after, I received thousands of emails and letters from around the world. Some were from readers who had been abused as children and, having found comfort in my books, wanted to share their own stories with me. I often felt truly humbled by their courage – the strength that had allowed them to put their suffering behind them and make a success of their lives. However, although many of these adults had managed to move on from the cruelty of the past – having successful careers, enjoying loving long-term relationships and raising children – others had not.

While I truly sympathized with their ongoing pain, I began to wonder why some survivors of abuse had managed to move on with their lives and others, years later, were still suffering, stuck in a really cruel and frightening place of depression, flashbacks, mental illness, suicide attempts, personality disorders, nightmares and self-harm. Was it just luck, I wondered, that had allowed some people to overcome their suffering and achieve happiness and contentment? Or were there other factors – for example, the extent of the abuse or the amount of time that had elapsed since? I discovered it was nothing like this.

As the emails continued to pour in I also heard from readers who confided that they were unhappy with their lives for no good reason. *Having read your books I know I should be grateful for my life but I seem to be fed up, bad tempered and down most of the time* was typical of many of these emails.

So what was it? I wondered. What magic wand had been waved over some people's lives to grant them happiness and contentment, and was this magic available to everyone? Could we all benefit? For even if we haven't suffered, life can sometimes seem an uphill struggle.

The answer I discovered was yes: there was a magic being worked and it could be available to all. So I began to look more closely to find a way to harness it.

I was soon able to tell from the opening lines of a letter or email into which category a person fell. Something in their language, their positivity or lack of it, said they were happy and contented with life, or the opposite. As the correspondence grew I began to see common threads appearing – in attitude and way of life. The magic was something that often the person was not even consciously aware of but had intuitively stumbled on and followed. So I extracted all the bits that had been proved to work and came up with *Happy Adults*: a formula for guaranteeing happiness and contentment.

Happy Adults

CHAPTER ONE

Let Go of Anger

Being angry – at ourselves or others – is responsible for the vast majority of our negative behaviour and feelings. While feeling anger and then letting it go is good for our mental health, hanging on to anger past its 'use by' date, or internalizing anger, can produce or aggravate all manner of physical and psychological illnesses – from stomach ulcers and migraines to severe psychosis. There is even evidence to suggest that cancer is more prevalent in people with angry negative dispositions than calmer more positive people, such is the interaction between mind and body.

Having said that, you do have the right to feel angry sometimes, and in some situations it is appropriate and healthy to do so.

It is right to feel angry if you accidentally hurt yourself – for example, cutting your finger while opening a can of beans. *Ouch! That hurt! How stupid of me!* Then the pain subsides and you let go of the anger and continue with what you were doing.

It is right to feel angry if someone treats you unfairly or unkindly – for example, your boss is highly critical of you in front of a less senior member of staff. Or a less able colleague is promoted over you. *How dare he treat me like that!*

You will feel angry if you discover a close friend and trusted confidante has been criticizing you behind your back. *Wait till I see him! I'll show him what I think of him!*

You will feel anger (and sorrow) if a loved one dies prematurely. *It's not fair: my mum was only thirty-nine. Why did she have to die and leave me?*

You will feel angry (and vulnerable) if someone has harmed you – physically or mentally. *I didn't do anything to him. Why me?*

It is appropriate to feel angry in all the above situations (and many others like them which crop up as part of normal life), but it is essential to know when to let go of the anger. While no one is likely to still be angry a month after cutting his or her finger on a tin, many of us can still be seething from being humiliated in front of a work colleague or gossiped about by a friend months, even years, after the event. But holding on to anger in this way will gnaw away at your confidence and self-esteem, making you depressed and bitter.

Compare these two extracts from readers' emails. They are both talking about their mothers.

> *I'll never forgive her as long as I live. Although she only lives three miles away I haven't seen her in nearly twenty years. I won't have her near my house. My brother sees her so I don't see him either. I have no family.* Ms A.

> *I wasn't going to let her ruin my life so I told her I still didn't understand why she hadn't believed me, but I was willing to move on. She now visits and sees her grandchildren. They love her dearly.* Ms B.

Both of these emails were from women in their mid-thirties. Both had been sexually abused as teenagers by their stepfathers. Both had told their mothers at the time what was happening and neither had been believed. Which of the two had the happier life? The second writer, Ms B. She had instinctively recognized that to hang on to her anger would 'ruin my life'. She was able to tell her mother that while she would never understand why she hadn't believed her when she'd told her she was being assaulted, she wanted to put the past behind them. By letting go of her anger, not only was Ms B more contented and happier but she had allowed her children to enjoy a relationship with their grandmother which they wouldn't otherwise have had.

Whether we have a very big anger – for example, as a result of being abused – or a relatively small anger – for example, a hurtful remark – at some point **we have to let go.** I am not being dismissive of the shocking suffering some people go through, but after an appropriate time (possibly with the help of therapy) we have to make a decision to let go of the anger, for if we don't we will stay trapped in misery, bitterness and self-loathing, and that will affect those around us. Ms A unfortunately had not been able to let go of her anger and was addicted to antidepressants, having had two failed marriages, and a daughter with whom she battled continuously. Anger and depression go hand in hand and are a result of our feelings of helplessness and despair. We have to let go of anger to allow ourselves to heal and depression to lift.

We therefore owe it to ourselves to let go of our anger, and to those around us too. Let me show you how.

The turning point

. . . .

I was furious when my husband, John, left me for a much younger woman. I was seething, not only for myself but on behalf of my children. How could he! How dare he! What a shit! How was I going to manage alone and provide for my family? My anger was with me for most of my waking days and at night, when, unable to sleep, I lay awake, tormented by thoughts of John and what he was doing in his new life.

I took my revenge. I unpicked the seams of his trousers, which still hung in the wardrobe and which he intended collecting when he had the time. I gave his collection of CDs to the charity shop and followed this with many other trips whenever I discovered an item of his he hadn't packed in his hasty departure. When his sister (with whom I'd always got on well) phoned to say she was sorry to hear John and I were having difficulties in our marriage and she hoped we could sort things out, I vented my anger on her. John had omitted to tell her the reason we were 'having difficulties' – that he had run off with a younger woman – but I had no difficulty in telling his sister, in vengeful graphic detail. I also said that I supposed I shouldn't be surprised John had deserted me, as clearly lack of commitment ran in his family. This was really nasty, as his sister had recently separated from her husband, but I was so angry I wanted to hurt everyone connected with him.

I said and did things which I would never normally have done and which now make me cringe with embarrassment. However, I stopped short of using the children against John. He saw them regularly and I didn't criticize him to the children, although I dearly wanted to.

I knew I had the right to be angry. I'd trusted John, believed what he'd told me and assumed we would stay married and raise our children together, as my parents had done. I was the innocent victim and my anger was appropriate, acceptable and a healthy outlet for my emotion at that time. But two years later when I was still too angry to give John the divorce he desperately wanted – by then his partner was pregnant and he wanted to marry her – my anger was no longer healthy or helpful. Indeed it was working against me. I had lost weight, taken up smoking again and stopped going out socially unless it was for the children. If anyone asked how I was (expecting to hear my divorce had been finalized and that I was ready to move on with my life) I lapsed again into the all-too-familiar lament of John's dreadful behaviour. I had become a martyr to his actions, a slave to his wrongdoing: my anger was now well past its 'use by' date and had turned sour.

Then one morning, two years after John had left me, I was brushing my hair in the mirror and caught sight of the woman I had become – still full of pain, suffering and anger. At that moment I knew I had to do something and quickly. I found myself giving that woman in the mirror a good talking to. My opening words changed my life and set me on the path to recovery. I said simply but firmly: *You have to admit your marriage is over. John has left you and is not coming back.* Though that was already apparent to many, part of me still thought he would return. I continued by telling myself: *Your future will be different – not the one you planned – but it can be a very good future. You have the most precious gift in the world: your children. Stop wallowing in self-pity and let go of your anger.*

> *Concentrate on all the positives in your life and move on. You owe it to you and you owe it to your children. It's time to stop being angry.*

I agree my words were not the most insightful, and the message they contained was probably obvious; however, it hadn't been obvious to me. I couldn't let go of my anger because I was still hankering after a life that could no longer be, and that anger was tainting all that was positive in my life. The 'good talking to' I gave myself was the **turning point.**

Likewise it had been for thousands of the readers who had emailed me with their experiences. The phrases *So I gave myself a good talking to* ... or *I told myself that* ... or *I said out loud I had to* ... came up time and time again. And, my readers told me, they had turned from anger, bitterness and depression to happiness and contentment. So the first step to letting go of your anger is to give yourself a 'good talking to'. In addressing yourself you are addressing your anger – the anger that has been making you unhappy for a long time.

When exactly the turning point arrives varies. It may come at the end of days, weeks or years of being angry. Clearly big hurts need longer to heal than smaller hurts, and while you are healing anger is acceptable and healthy. But you will know when your anger is past its 'use by' date. You will know when it is time to let go and move on, and when it is time look at yourself in the mirror and address yourself honestly.

Remember it doesn't have to be a big hurt that is making you angry and unhappy. Even if you are angry about a small hurt, at some point you have to let go. In a lifetime we have to let go of anger many, many times, for life is full of situations which cause us pain and suffering, and if left unaddressed the anger and resentment fester, making us unhappy and depressed.

Here are a few more examples of the turning point:

I can still remember being unjustly accused by my departmental manager of being late on my third day at work (my first job) at the age of eighteen. I was in fact at work but attending a training session in another room, which my manager hadn't been informed of. The manager shouted at me in front of the whole office before I had a chance to explain. I can still remember my feelings of humiliation and anger and wishing the ground would open up and swallow me. Looking back, I can see that the man may have been a bully, but it is true to say that the scene ruined my first months at work. I inwardly seethed, from both the injustice and the humiliation. My spirits sank to the point where I considered handing in my notice. Monday mornings were a nightmare.

Then I made a conscious decision to address myself: *It was a silly thing for him to say but I am not responsible for his actions. We've got on well until now. I will not hold it against him any more.* I let go of my anger and focused on all the good things about the job, of which there were many. It was a conscious decision, as letting go of anger often has to be, and once I'd let go of my anger my spirits lifted, I began to enjoy the work and the incident took its rightful place in history.

A nineteen-year-old rape victim whose attacker had not been prosecuted because of a technicality in the law was consumed by anger at the injustice (understandably). But it was dominating her life and she was blaming herself. She wrote that she had found her turning point by addressing herself as follows: *I am so angry he wasn't prosecuted. He should have been. I did all I could, but it wasn't my decision. It was the police who decided not to prosecute. I had no control over that decision but I do have control over the rest of my life. I'm not going to let him ruin it.*

A woman of thirty-two wrote about her mother who had given her other daughter (the writer's sister) a diamond ring that she had inherited from her mother and had sentimental value. The woman had seen the favouritism and had translated it as her mother loving her sister more than she loved her. She had been upset and angry for over a year and this anger was souring her relationship with her mother and sister, whom she loved dearly. The turning point for her came when she addressed herself as follows: *My mother decided to give that ring to my sister. It was her choice. Although it's going to be very difficult, I need to stop being angry and ask her why she decided to do that. Have I done something to upset her?*

When she finally plucked up the courage to ask her mother, she wished she'd asked her sooner and so avoided a year of anger, pain and resentment. Her mother's actions were entirely innocent of any favouritism. It was simply that the other daughter had always been fascinated by the ring, right from childhood, so when the ring no longer fitted the mother's finger (because of arthritis) she had naturally given it to the daughter who had been interested in it, never dreaming she was causing her other daughter pain. The mother apologized, although there was no need, for the writer knew what her mother was saying was true.

Perhaps what has caused you to be angry and depressed is not one incident but a culmination of small incidents that have built up over time. Or it may be there aren't any incidents at all, but just an ongoing gnawing anger that life promised you something and hasn't delivered.

One reader from the US wrote: *I was fed up with my life; nothing seemed right. There was no reason. I mean I hadn't been abused like the children in your books but there didn't seem any point to life. I was twenty-nine and hooked on antidepressants and pills to make me sleep. I really hated the person I had become – negative, angry and finding fault in everything. It's a wonder I had any friends left at all. Then one evening after a really bad day I asked myself: do you really want to carry on like this or are you going to try and find something better? I realized at that moment it was down to*

me: my future was in my hands. I could carry on as I was –
unhappy and hating everything – or I could change and be
happy.

The woman carried on to say that with the help of a
life coach, who showed her how to focus on the positives in life, she had stopped taking all the pills and was
finally enjoying life.

Whatever the reason, if you are angry you will be unhappy
and at some point you need to make a conscious decision
to let go and move on. For this woman the turning point
was the question *Do you really want to carry on like this*, her
acknowledgement that she didn't and her readiness to
move on and do something different. It may help to say out
loud why it's time to let go. In my case it was *You have to
admit your marriage is over.*

We can sometimes take on responsibility for the actions
of others, convincing ourselves we are to blame for the
outcome when in fact we have no control of those actions,
and this results in us feeling frustrated and angry. In such
cases we need to pass the responsibility for the bad word or
deed back to the person who had issued it, acknowledging
their responsibility (as in the case of the rape victim, where
she acknowledged that it was the police's decision not to
prosecute) or if necessary asking that person why they
acted as they had, before we can let go of our anger and
move on.

You may find you need some extra help to move on, as
the lady who approached a life coach did. Don't be afraid to

ask for help, from whichever source you feel most comfortable with – a counsellor, a life coach, a therapist, your minister, your guardian angel or your god. You have made the decision to move on; if you need extra help, take it.

When you reach the turning point, you can take action by acknowledging the truth, thereby allowing yourself to deal with the anger and move on to happiness and contentment.

CHAPTER TWO

·····································

Take Responsibility for Your Life

While we are not responsible for the decisions and actions of others (as we saw in the last chapter) **we are always responsible for our own decisions and actions**, although sometimes we would rather not admit it.

> *If he had shown me more affection I wouldn't have needed an affair …*

> *She went on at me until I hit her. She should have left it. I can go out with my mates if I want.*

These two readers were trying to transfer blame and therefore responsibility to their partners. On occasions we are all guilty of blaming others for our actions and the reason we do so is obvious. *If only he/she hadn't I wouldn't have … They shouldn't have put temptation in my way ….* etc. Transferring the blame, in our eyes, transfers the responsibility and therefore lets us off, or so we would like to believe. Clearly this is untrue, for we are only transferring the responsibility in our minds. No one else has accepted responsibility for our actions. We haven't been let off the hook: we are simply in denial.

> A man aged forty-three wrote: *I blame my father for always criticizing me as a child. I couldn't do anything right. If I got a B grade he said I should have got an A. If I scored a goal he asked me why I'd missed the other two shots.* The man wrote that in adult life he reacted very badly if he thought anyone was criticizing him, becoming angry and aggressive, even when the criticism was in fact constructive feedback from his boss at work. He knew he was over-sensitive to what he perceived as criticism and his reaction was causing a problem both at work and in his private life. His wife felt she was 'walking on egg shells' and daren't say anything in case he took it personally.

From what the man said it was likely his father had been over-critical, but by using his father as a convenient scape-goat for any negatives in his life, and failing to take responsibility for his own failings, he was endangering his relationships at home and work. I have been taken aback by the number of other readers in middle age and older who are still able to blame their parents (or carers) for all that was wrong in their present lives. No parent is perfect; parents are fallible human beings and will get their parenting wrong as often as they get it right. Without doubt some people have easier and happier childhoods than others, but as adults we owe it to ourselves to **take responsibility** for the present and future and move on. As a general guideline, if you haven't taken responsibility for your own life by the age of twenty-five, then you need to do so ASAP. Otherwise life will be a series of missed opportunities, regrets, discontent and unhappiness. While we can't change the past, by taking responsibility we can change the present and future. **The key to our success is entirely in our own hands.**

As well as blaming others and assigning to them responsibility for our lives, we are also very good at blaming situations, circumstances and even fate. *I know I'm not being offered the jobs because of my size*, wrote one reader who was in her mid-twenties and weighed 25 stone. Her CV was excellent and she was readily called for interview for jobs as a receptionist. But as soon as she walked into the interview room, she said, she knew from the look on the interviewers' faces that she wouldn't be offered the job. There is a lot of prejudice towards large people which won't change overnight. The harsh reality is that if the woman wants a job as a receptionist she is going to have to take responsibility and diet, or accept that she must look for a job where her appearance doesn't have to conform to a norm.

A lad of eighteen who had failed his exams and dropped out of school wrote: *I have a big family with six stepbrothers and sisters. There was never anywhere that was quiet for me to study. That's why I failed.* He was bemoaning being unemployed and having no money. I appreciated that it must have been difficult for him to study at home, but if he had taken responsibility he could have found somewhere quiet to study, such as the library or homework club at school. Even though he now recognized he needed qualifications to get a job, he was still refusing to take responsibility. One option would have been to enrol in a college course to gain the qualifications he needed, and his mother had suggested this, but the lad had a ready list of excuses as to why this or any other suggestion wouldn't work. Until he took responsibility for his life he was going to continue disgruntled and without a job.

A woman, aged forty-five, who had been in foster care for a year at the age of eight, wrote that she blamed all that was currently wrong in her life, including her two sons being drug dependent, her husband's domestic violence and her obesity, on being in care thirty-seven years previously. While I would never minimize the disruption being taken into care (or any other trauma over which a person has no control) can have on a young person's life, by allowing a crisis in her past to become a convenient peg on which to hang responsibility for all her woes and misfortunes, this woman was not taking any responsibility for them herself.

Whether we are suffering as a result of an unhappy/ abusive childhood, losing a job, a hurtful comment or action, a failed relationship or a divorce, bereavement, ill health or a fateful encounter, at some point we have to take responsibility for our lives and deal with whatever needs to be changed. Otherwise we are like flotsam on a wave – sloshed around at the will of the tide and never in control of our destiny.

A man, aged twenty-three, who drank excessively and drove while intoxicated, was stopped by the police, heavily fined and banned from driving for two years. He was then sacked from his job, which required a clean driving licence. He blamed fate and an old friend: *If I hadn't stopped off at that pub after work I wouldn't have met him and none of this would have happened.* A better response, where the man took responsibility, would have been: *What an idiot I was! But I've learnt my lesson. When I get my licence back I'll never drink and drive again. In the meantime I'll have to find a job for which I don't need a driving licence.*

Taking responsibility for your life is fantastic! It puts you at the steering wheel and you can go wherever you want. Yes, it can appear a bit frightening before you begin your journey. But once you have assumed responsibility for your life and therefore your destiny, you'll wonder how you ever managed before.

What you gain from taking responsibility

Let's look at all the positive outcomes from taking responsibility for your life; there are no negatives!

1. Empowerment. Taking responsibility empowers you. Once you are in charge you can do anything you wish – even fly to the moon, as long as you train as an astronaut first. You decide what you want to do with your life – where you want to be in a week, a month, a year, ten years – and go for it. Many years ago when I was struggling as a writer, receiving more rejection slips than cheques, I was inspired by the maxim *We are only limited by the extent of our imagination*. It is so true, and by taking responsibility we empower ourselves to achieve whatever our hearts and minds desire.

2. Liberation. Taking responsibility liberates you from the constraints of others. If you pass responsibility for your life to others you will live in the shadow of their experiences, expectations, successes and failures, and this will result in you becoming frustrated and discontented. Once you take responsibility for your life you are no longer beholden to the actions, attitudes or opinions of others, and a huge burden lifts from your shoulders.

> One woman, aged thirty-four, who was juggling family life with work and doing unpaid overtime until 6.15 most nights, felt she was 'being used' and a 'slave' to everyone else, although she knew her husband loved her. She wrote: *So I finally stopped blaming everyone else for what was wrong with my life and decided to take responsibility. I explained to my boss (nicely) that I would be leaving at 5.30 in future as I had family commitments. To my surprise he was fine about it, and said he understood and that I should have said something sooner. I then had a big chat with my husband and said I needed some 'me time'. I am now having*

ice-skating lessons – something I always wanted to do – on a Wednesday evening, while my husband looks after the children. I was surprised it was all so easy in the end. I felt a great sense of liberation. I am in control of my life again and I'm sure I'm a much nicer person to be with now, at home and work.

3. Achievement. When you take responsibility for your life you can also take the credit for your achievements. What a great bonus! Yes, you may be working alongside others on certain projects and your relationships will be a partnership, but whether you are working on something alone, with someone else, or in a group, any positive outcome you achieve is your responsibility. So give yourself a big pat on the back.

4. Development. By taking responsibility for your life you develop as a person. You learn from your mistakes and use your past experiences to make better judgements in the future. Each new decision you make – regardless of how small or disastrous the outcome – is character forming. You will develop a strength and roundness of character you never thought possible. Others will experience and appreciate your new-found inner strength, although they won't necessarily recognize the transition you have made. Your development as a person and therefore your new resourcefulness of character will be magnetic. Very soon you will be one of those people others come to for advice and guidance.

5. Satisfaction and contentment. Taking responsibility for your life allows you the satisfaction and contentment of knowing you did your best. Even if the outcome is not as you had hoped, knowing you were in control and you couldn't have done any more gives you peace of mind.

CHAPTER THREE

Think Positively

We are what we think. Consider this statement for a moment and its implications. How far reaching it is; how simple; how complex; how easy and yet unobtainable!

'We are what we think' means that our thoughts create the person we are now and will be in the future. Just as our bodies absorb food and we become what we eat (I say more about this on page 60), so our personalities are a product of what we think. Our thoughts govern who we are and therefore our actions, which clearly influence our future. Research has also shown that our state of mind directly influences our bodies.

We are all familiar with the scenario of 'getting out of the wrong side of the bed'. Not literally, of course, but that feeling at the start of a new day that we are full of self-doubt and pessimism and at odds with the world. We know what type of day we are going to have – one when we wished we'd stayed in bed. It will be a day when others and situations seem to conspire against us, when we achieve little or nothing, and hostility and aggravation are all around us. On such a day we get exactly what we envisaged, and as a result we feel unhappy and discontented.

We are also familiar with the opposite scenario, when we start the new day full of optimism. Our thoughts and feelings are positive: we focus on what is right in our lives and we are more than ready to greet any new challenge. We are so full of positive thoughts and vibes that we can't have anything but a good day – we achieve what we set out to and others appear to work with us and are on our side. We feel good about ourselves and are happy to be alive.

Then of course there are the days in the middle of the spectrum when we greet the new day with ambivalence, not particularly enthusiastic about what lies ahead but not dreading it. The day holds no surprises, we get by – achieving an acceptable amount, jogging along but not really engaging with those we come in contact with. If someone were to ask us: *Have you had a good day?* We would reply: *It was OK.*

In reality these three days were probably no different from each other in their happiness content. Happiness content means the external factors, negative and positive, that directly affect our happiness – for example, a pay rise, the birth of a child, the death of a loved one, marriage, divorce, etc. No, what made each of these days different was literally our state of mind: our attitude, based on our positive or negative thoughts.

As the optimist sees the glass as half full, so the pessimist sees it as half empty. The only difference between the two is the way they think.

A person in a positive state of mind who is thinking positive thoughts expects to be happy, achieve and get along with those he or she meets, while a person in a negative state of mind can see only gloom, despondency, non-cooperation and frustration, with little or nothing achieved. These two people will have their positive or negative attitude confirmed by getting exactly what they expect. This is what is known as a 'self-fulfilling prophecy', where something we perceive in our minds becomes true because of the link between belief and behaviour. **If we think positively then we act positively, which leads to a positive outcome. Conversely, negative thoughts produce negative actions and outcomes.**

Positive and negative thoughts are like magnets, attracting those in a similar state of mind. So a person in positive frame of mind will attract positive, happy people, who add to his or her feel-good factor, and 'repel' negative ones. Conversely a person in a negative state of mind will be a magnet for the negativity of others, who will collude in his or her feelings of self-doubt and pessimism. Of course, this takes place subconsciously, with each person acting instinctively, without conscious thought or decision.

Since all this has a huge impact on our lives on all levels, mental and physical, we owe it to ourselves to think positively. It is essential we recognize and harness the incredible power of the mind to achieve mental and physical well-being.

Many ancient cultures were aware of the power of the mind and its effect on physical health. The age-old practice of yoga is a physical and mental discipline whose purpose includes physical health. Likewise meditation is an intrinsic part of many ancient healings, as is the Chinese philosophy of yin and yang, which acknowledges the need to find the right balance.

But while such cultures acknowledge that the mind and body are interconnected, many Western cultures, especially with the advancement in medical science, separate mind and body, with disastrous results. We have blood, nerves and energy lines running through and linking all parts of ourselves, mind and body. Why, then, do we treat them separately, having one branch of medicine for the body – GPs, medical consultants and surgeons – and another for our minds – psychiatrists, therapists and counsellors? In recent years there has been some movement in Western culture towards a more holistic approach – that is, treating the whole person – but it still has a long way to go.

The good news, however, is that we can change the way we think. Positive thought is within our control. We can choose to think positively, which will improve the person we are now and ultimately what happens in our lives.

Positive thought is straightforward and easy to learn, but it won't happen overnight. Like all strategies it needs to be learnt until it becomes second nature and you do it automatically. This is what you do to achieve it.

How to think positively

1. Focus on all that is good in your life and the world around you. Acknowledge the negative but don't dwell on it. If you find your thoughts returning to the negative, rein them in and re-focus. This gets easier the more you do it.

2. Focus on your attributes. You have much to offer. Acknowledge your failings and weaknesses but don't dwell on them. None of us is perfect.

3. Visualize positive outcomes. Research has shown that if you believe something will turn out well you increase the chances of it doing so.

4. Think good of others. See the best in other people; give them the benefit of the doubt, don't harbour grudges, forgive them and move on (see Chapter One).

5. Be grateful. Even the most disadvantaged of us has something to be grateful for. Recognize it and be thankful it is yours.

6. Get rid of the belief that life owes you. It doesn't. The only person who owes is you and you owe it to yourself to make the best of life.

To do this, you need to be aware of what is happening in your thoughts. During the day our thought processes vary to accommodate what we are doing: reading or studying, at work, being on the computer, watching television, listening to music, engaging in conversation, concentrating on a difficult task, relaxing, etc. Sometimes our thoughts will be wholly occupied by what we are doing, but at other times there is space for our thoughts to cruise or wander. It is at such times, when we are off guard, not wholly concentrating, that we are most likely to find ourselves thinking negative thoughts if we are in a negative state of mind: *I hate him. My nose is too big. Why did she cheat on me? There can't be a God: he wouldn't have let my mum die so young* and so on.

Be aware of your thoughts and deal with any negativity immediately. Don't indulge this negativity; instead, acknowledge your feelings, and then let go of them and consciously shift your mind to a positive thought. By using this strategy of counteracting a negative thought with a positive thought you can retrain your mind.

I think my nose is too big (negative), *but people tell me I have nice eyes and a pleasant smile, which is good* (positive).

I hate him for what he did to me (negative), *but that part of my life is over now and I have a great future ahead of me* (positive).

I don't know why she cheated on me (negative), *but it's just as well I found out now rather than later* (positive).

I wish my mum was still alive (negative); *I miss her dread-fully. But thank God she was my mum and we had all those good years together. Some people don't have that* (positive).

You can find something positive in virtually every negative situation, even when the situation is dreadful. I am sure we were all impressed by the young soldier who, having lost both his legs and one arm when a landmine exploded, said in an interview that it could have been worse, and at least he still had one arm. Or the countless number of cancer sufferers who, having been told they only have a short while to live, decide to make the most of every minute, focusing on the days they have left rather than the years they have been deprived.

While you are retraining your mind to think positively there will be times when you slip into your old way of thinking. As soon as you catch yourself doing this, whether it is on waking, showering, eating, dressing, sitting on a train, playing with the children or at work, acknowledge your negative thoughts and make the next thought positive. It is important to acknowledge the negative thought: otherwise it can be buried without being dealt with and you can go into denial. All feelings are important, but negative thinkers focus on what is wrong in their lives to the exclusion of all that is right. If your mind returns to the negative, bring it back again to a positive thought. Soon this will become second nature, and hey presto, you will be a positive thinker!

I am a positive thinker but I haven't always been. As a teenager I used to dwell on all the sadness in the world (over which I had no control) and make myself very unhappy. Positive thinking came to me in my twenties, after a traumatic experience, and has been my companion ever since. It sees me through life's downers and makes me appreciate every new day.

The children I foster often arrive depressed and unhappy – with very good reason: they have been separated from their families and have often been abused or badly neglected. By the time they leave me all of them are a lot, lot happier. While I haven't been able to change their family situation or their past experience (unfortunately), I have been able to help them towards an acceptance of what has happened, and encourage them to think positively and this helps them to see a positive, brighter future.

Young children and even toddlers can be encouraged to think positively as soon as they begin taking an interest in their surroundings. There is beauty everywhere; sometimes we just need to see it. By pointing out the little robin in your garden, or the clear blue sky, or asking your child if he or she is enjoying their ice cream – 'Mmm, that looks yummy. I bet it tastes good' – you are encouraging your child to think positively.

One woman wrote: *I spent over twenty years thinking about all that was wrong in my life (and believe me there was plenty). I thought life wasn't fair as others didn't seem to*

have my problems. I made myself so miserable I even consid-
ered suicide. Then one day I was in the dentist's waiting room
and picked up a copy of an old magazine. In it was an article
about positive thinking and that article changed my life.

The notion of positive thinking is not new, but when you discover its huge power and the possibilities it opens up for happiness and contentment it seems like a revelation. It is life changing!

CHAPTER FOUR

Act Positively

Thinking positively, however, is only part of the equation that is lasting happiness and contentment. To feel the full benefit of a positive state of mind, you need to put your positive thoughts into action. **Positive people are doers, positive in thought and action.** They attract other positive people and together they make things happen.

The next piece of good news is that once you are using the power of positive thinking, acting positively is only a small step away.

Positive action follows positive thought. If you have started thinking positively you may already be practising some of the following strategies, without even realizing it, which is great. Read through the following, congratulate yourself on what you are already doing and take on board the areas you still need to work on. As with positive thinking, to begin with you will have to make a conscious effort to act positively, but very soon it will become automatic, with the result that you are both thinking and acting positively – a truly positive person.

How to act positively

1. Smile. As often as you can. If smiling doesn't come naturally to you, force yourself to smile to begin with until it does. Research has shown that smiling has a natural feel-good factor. It releases endorphins (natural painkillers) and serotonin (sometimes called the body's natural opium) into the bloodstream, literally making you happy. When you smile the facial muscles send messages of happiness to the brain, and you feel happy. Even when you are feeling unhappy, **smiling can make you happy.** Also, research trials have shown that when you smile others perceive you differently – as younger, more confident, successful and attractive. Smiling has been shown to relieve stress by lowering blood pressure, and also to strengthen the immune system. Happy, positive people are ill less often. Smiling is therefore beneficial on all levels and is an essential ingredient to being positive. So smile away.

2. Try new things. Set yourself realistic goals – short and long term – and do your very best to achieve them. (I'll say more about this in Chapter Six.) If you've been wanting to learn a new skill, try a new hobby or even change your lifestyle or career, then do it. Don't be frightened to try something new, whether it is swimming, skating, camping, debating, cake decorating, joining a political party or volunteering. All new experiences add to being a positive person. Our confidence and self-esteem grow from experiencing new challenges, and who knows where such new experience might lead?

One woman wrote: *I was feeling pretty miserable as my fiftieth birthday approached. I was overweight and despite dieting couldn't seem to shift the flab. My husband bought me a pair of quality trainers for a birthday present as I said I might try jogging. On that first morning I could barely run round the block, I was red in the face and panting, but I kept with it. Gradually my stamina built and the weight dropped off. Now I compete in marathons all over the world. I feel so fit and have made many new friends. Jogging has opened up a whole new life for me and I know my husband is proud of me. He claims it was the trainers that did it, but I say they couldn't have done it without me!*

A man who went fishing caught more than he could ever have dreamed of: *I'd always wanted to learn to fish, right from a boy, so at the ripe old age of forty-two I bought myself a fishing rod and all the gear, and early one Sunday morning I left my wife and kids in bed and went and sat by a local river. It was pouring down and there was only me and a couple of lads, which I was pleased about, as I was making a fool of myself trying to cast the line.*

Then a guy came along and said he was a journalist from the local newspaper and he was writing an article about local fishing spots and would I mind if he took a photo of me? I told him it was my first fishing trip but he said that was fine as I looked the part. A week later the photo was published in our local newspaper with my name, and an article about fishing spots. I looked very professional with all my new gear although all I'd caught that morning was a cold.

Then a few weeks later I received a letter forwarded to me by the newspaper. When I opened it I was amazed to find it was from my long-lost brother, whom I hadn't seen for fifteen years. He'd seen my photo in the paper, and it turned out he only lived a mile away. We met up and I discovered he was a keen (and very good) fisherman. So now I go fishing with my brother while our wives go shopping.

Both these people changed their lives in ways they couldn't have envisaged by trying something new. That's not to say you'll become a globetrotter if you take up jogging, or find a brother if you go fishing, but one thing is for certain: life doesn't happen in front of the television or at the computer. Experience happens in the real world and positive people make it happen by going out and trying new things.

3. Use positive words as much as possible when speaking about yourself, others or situations:

I consider myself a fair person …

John is very patient …

It was decent of our company to still give us the bonus when profits are down, even though it was smaller than last year's.

Even if you have a highly critical report to deliver, include as many positive words as you can. And generally, when you speak make sure you use more positive than negative words. I often have to talk at meetings about children who have severe behavioural problems, and I always begin my report with all the positives, which sets the atmosphere for the meeting. There is something positive in every person and situation; find it and say it. Whether you are talking casually to a friend or relative, or formally in a meeting at work, feast on the positive and acknowledge but don't dwell on the negative.

4. Give praise where it is due. It won't detract from your own worth to acknowledge what others have achieved. Praise is not a bag of sweets where the quantity diminishes as you share them out: it is more like fresh air – free and plentiful. As an author I have met some authors who are loathe to speak highly of their colleagues (especially if they are writing in the same genre), because of some misguided notion that praising others will detract from their own success. Of course it doesn't; if anything it has the opposite effect. In praising others we show we are comfortable in our role, and insightful enough as a person to recognize and admire achievement.

Mark, that was an excellent report. Thanks for your input. I really appreciated it.

Mum, you are a smashing grandma. You have so much patience. The kids love you to bits.

Jane, that dress looks far better on you than it ever did on me. You have it.

What a great job you did decorating the sitting room!

Praise and positive feedback cost you nothing but have a huge effect on the recipient and yourself. **Praise is like a kiss to the soul:** we feel warm and glow from the approval of others. Not only does it make us feel good about ourselves but we also feel good about the person who praised us. We warm to that person and unsurprisingly research has shown that we bond more quickly with those who give praise and positive feedback than with those who remain neutral – not criticizing but not saying anything positive either.

Give yourself a quiet pat on the back, too, for something you have achieved, but keep self-praise to yourself unless you say it light-heartedly:

I think I did a good job there, don't you, lads?

Job well done!

Didn't she do well! (referring to yourself)

Leave effusive praise of yourself to others. No one likes a big head.

5. Make friends and reach out to people. We need friends as much as we need family. Framed on a wall in my home is a piece of embroidery given to me by my grandmother. It is made up of hundreds of tiny cross-stitches and states, quite simply, 'A Family is a Circle of Friends Who Love You'. I've treasured this for years; the words are so poignant and have meaning on many levels. I even used the words to start a group on the social networking site Facebook.

Even if you are a naturally shy person, when you are thinking and acting more positively you will be in a much better position to meet new people and make friends. Begin with the smile you've been practising; then offer a small remark (in the UK the weather is a safe bet); then, if the situation allows, follow this initial contact with conversation. Not everyone you meet will become a lasting friend, but just reaching out and making contact with others – whether it is at the bus stop, at the supermarket checkout or in the lift at work – boosts our confidence and feelings of self-worth. Even grumbling with others at a bus stop about the bus being late is positive: it releases our frustration and bonds us with others in the same situation – the 'pack', as social scientists call it. Humans have always lived in groups and we need that sense of belonging as much now as we did when we lived in caves and hunted as a pack.

6. Learn to say no. Don't be a martyr. Acting positively doesn't mean you always have to agree to all the requests that are made of you. Far from it. Although positive people reach out and interact with others easily they also know how to give a polite refusal. No one likes a martyr who glories in suffering from too much to do. Such a person makes us lesser mortals feel very uncomfortable. We need to self-regulate the responsibilities and workload we accept. I developed the art of saying no many years ago when I realized that fostering, as well as raising my own children and working part-time, did not allow me to help in fund-raising activities or sit on the PTA at my children's school or do many of the other things I was asked to do. Agree to do what you can and want to do, and politely refuse what you don't want to do or can't do without causing yourself stress:

I'm sorry, I really can't continue on the Neighbourhood Watch scheme as I am heavily committed with other projects.

I'm sorry, Mary, I won't be able to look after your children on Saturday as John and I are decorating the living room.

Bob, could you give Susie that report to type, please? I'm up to my eyes in it at present. Thanks.

If you find that in your role at home or work your stress levels are continually rising as you run to stand still, then you are over-committed and you need to have a discussion with your boss or partner. If you soldier on without saying anything others will assume you are coping. Positive people recognize their limitations and can say no.

7. Be body positive. I say more about this in Chapter Eight. But it is worth noting here that when you are thinking and acting more positively your body language should reflect this so that you present your new improved self to the world. So often our bodies get left behind after radical change: the body carries on as it used to, as it has been doing for years. Dieters who lose a lot of weight, for instance, often need lessons in deportment, to be shown how to walk gracefully. Their new, lighter, sylph-like figures are still lumbering along as they did before when they carried all the extra weight.

Stand upright, look people in the eye and walk with a lighter, slightly faster step. The message you will give out is that you are confidently ready to meet and greet life and all it has to offer. Others will subconsciously receive your positive body signals and treat you accordingly.

CHAPTER FIVE

Develop a Positive Philosophy

We all have a philosophy – a system of beliefs that guide our behaviour – although we might not realize it. As humans we are programmed to make sense of what we see, from the moment we look up from our cribs and focus on the world around us. From then on we begin to develop a philosophy to make sense of the world and our existence in it.

The word philosophy in its academic sense means the study of knowledge, reality and existence. Western philosophy dates back over 2,500 years. During our time at school most of us will have heard of the ancient Greek philosophers – Plato, Socrates, Aristotle – and the more recent philosophers – Francis Bacon, Marx and Ghandi. Philosophers develop a way of thinking and looking at the world they hope will answer age-old questions such as *What is good? Do we have free will? Does God exist? What is truth? Where does infinity end? What is evil?* As individuals we contemplate these questions too and develop our personal philosophy to answer them.

While our philosophy reflects what we think about the world and our place in it, in practice, in our everyday lives, it is not a written tangible formula but the attitude with which we live our lives. Our philosophy is our outlook on life, shown in the way we deal with situations (past and present, negative and positive), view the future and make decisions. And if we are to be happy and contented and live life to the full, our philosophy needs to be positive.

Often our philosophy can be seen in the sayings we use, known as maxims or idioms. These sayings can be divided into three groups:

Positive maxims, suggesting the person has developed an optimistic view of life:

Every cloud has a silver lining.

Lightning never strikes twice in the same place.

When one door closes another opens.

The longest journey begins with the smallest step.

Things happen for a reason.

Negative maxims, suggesting cynicism, scepticism, mistrust and doubt, with the person expecting the worst-case scenario:

It's too good to be true.

It never rains but it pours.

You can't teach an old dog new tricks.

Butter wouldn't melt in his mouth.

Neutral maxims, where the phrase is a comment or observation:

You can't make an omelette without breaking eggs.

Never leave till tomorrow what you can do today.

A watched pot/kettle never boils.

A bird in the hand is worth two in the bush.

Actions speak louder than words.

Unsurprisingly, happy and contented people find them-selves using **positive maxims.** They believe a positive can be found in every situation and that positives far outweigh the negatives in life, and their philosophy – expressed in their maxims – reflects their belief system. A positive philosophy will see a person through the bad times, for they know the situation will improve because, on balance, they believe life is very good.

One woman wrote: *I knew I'd had my share of grief and that life would just get better and better. Ten years on I've been proved right: I have a job I love and a beautiful family of my own.* This was from a woman who had every reason to hate the world, having witnessed her father kill her mother.

And how I admire the boy, aged twelve, who wrote to me, having being bullied and taunted at school: *I knew if I let them [the bullies] see they had hurt me then they had won. So I walked away and I knew when the bell went at 3.20 I would have a good evening because my conscience was clear. They have to live with what they have done. I wouldn't want to be in their shoes.* My heart went out to him. What an intelligent, positive and courageous lad! I was sure he would do very well in life with his philosophy, although I encouraged him to report the bullies.

My philosophy can be best summed up as follows: Life is short and we never know what's around the corner, so I make the most of every day.

Because this is my outlook on life, I always look for the silver lining to any dark cloud and I know there is positive in any situation, no matter how dreadful. As a foster carer I hear the most awful accounts of children being abused, which could seriously undermine my faith in human nature and make me very depressed. To counteract this I see the incredible courage and resilience in the children them-selves and the huge improvements they make when they come into foster care. In addition, since I've had my fostering memoirs published, I've received thousands of emails from readers all around the world, sending their love, sharing their own stories, and giving me words of kindness and support. This confirms for me that the vast majority of people are intrinsically kind and the world is a good place.

I always try to pass on my philosophy to the children I look after, showing them the beauty around us and what makes life worth living, and encouraging them to live for the present and look forward to a better future. Even the saddest child can eventually find a glimmer of hope and start to leave the past behind. That glimmer may come in the call of a bird in spring; the early morning dew on a spider's web; the fiery orange sky as the sun sets in autumn; or the touch of a kind and caring hand.

Think about your own philosophy. Is it weighted in favour of the positive – optimism? Do you see the best in situations and people? Can you use your philosophy to deal with and dispel the negative and move on? If the answer is no, then you need to learn to think positively, as described in Chapter Three. To be happy and contented, your philosophy, your attitude to life, should not be *It never rains but it pours* or *It's too good to be true* but *Every cloud has a silver lining* or *When one door closes another opens*.

One last word (or rather two) before we leave the subject of philosophy: **be philosophical.** By that I mean use your (positive) philosophy to stay calm and manage challenging situations. So, for instance, if you bump your car, look at the damage, sigh and console yourself that the damage could have been worse. Or if you don't get an A grade in the exam you took, be philosophical and say, *Well, at least I passed!* If you didn't pass, then take heart that it isn't the end of the world and you can always take the exam again. There is positive in every situation, and being philosophical allows you to see and accept the positive, which leads to a brighter and happier way of life.

CHAPTER SIX

Set Goals and Have a Vision

Goals and a vision are essential for a happy and contented life. They are **always positive** and **give meaning, motivation and satisfaction** to our lives. Without goals or a vision we aim for little and achieve even less, dragging ourselves out of bed each morning to another day of repetition, boredom and drudgery, with little or no commitment.

Our goals are the aims, short and long term, that we **aspire to, work towards** and can reasonably **achieve.** Vision is slightly different. It is a long-term plan, a hope, a desire, something we have our sights set on, something that if our fairy godmother appeared we would ask her for. As well as having a personal vision most of us have a global vision – such as an end to war, famine greed and cruelty – which we take small steps to achieving, for example, through charity donations, voting in political leaders who reflect our beliefs, going on protest marches, etc. While realizing our global vision is largely outside our control, our personal vision is as attainable as our goals.

Goals

The goals we set for ourselves should be realistic – i.e. within our grasp. They may be personal to us or we may share them with a larger group, for example our family. Our goals, particularly our short-term goals, will change as we achieve them and move on to the next goal. Examples of personal **short-term goals** include:

* learning a new simple skill: for example, skating, badminton, tennis, swimming
* writing a report or finishing an essay
* painting a picture
* catching an earlier train to work so we are not late again
* cleaning out the rabbit hutch or taking the dog for a walk
* doing the housework
* being more patient with a demanding child
* saving a set amount each week or month, or clearing an overdraft.

Personal goals are the tasks we set ourselves on a daily, weekly or monthly basis. Often we set ourselves short-term goals and achieve them without even realizing it.

Long-term goals require more planning and forethought, so we are usually aware of their existence as we work towards attaining them. Long-term goals are bigger, more challenging, far reaching, and require more determination and effort, over months and even years. Examples include:

* studying for an exam, a degree or professional qualification
* decorating the house
* starting a family
* paying off the mortgage or moving house
* acquiring a new and complex skill such as learning a foreign language, learning to drive or learning to sign read
* walking the Great Wall of China
* writing a book
* becoming a manager, managing director, consultant, etc.

Group goals are the aims and ambitions of a group we belong to. The group may be our family, circle of friends, work colleagues, evening class or club we are a member of. The group will have short- and long-term goals which might be:

* saving for a special family holiday, moving house or emigrating
* starting up or expanding a business
* Parent Teachers Association (PTA) fundraising to build a swimming pool or gym for the school
* attaining promotion for the amateur football, rugby team, etc, you play for.

Some short-term goals will fall in the wider picture of our long-term goals. For example:

* researching for the essay you have to write to attain your degree
* saving for the flat you want to buy, or holiday you wish to go on
* shopping for the birthday party you're going to throw
* collecting data for the company's five-year plan.

Personal goals are essential for a positive, meaningful, happy and contented life because they give us purpose while we pursue them, and when we achieve them we feel satisfaction and accomplishment. With the achievement of long-term goals the feeling can be immense; we may even feel slightly deflated and aimless for a while, until we find the next goal to aim for.

Even in adverse circumstances it is still vital we set ourselves short- and long-term goals. If you are unemployed, for instance, setting short- and long-term goals including the routine of getting up at a reasonable time (as we did when we went to work), job hunting, speaking to friends, reading and acquiring new skills that will increase our chances of finding work. All of which will add to your positive feelings of self-worth, happiness and contentment.

When you achieve your goal, whether it is short- or long-term, personal or group, it is essential to congratulate yourself and enjoy the satisfaction and reward of what you have done. The achievement of short-term personal goals may easily be missed in the rush of everyday life, but it feels good and builds your confidence to recognize what you have gained, whether it is winning a contract at work or making a meal from a new recipe at home. So when you accomplish something, take a moment to give yourself a pat on the back, or if it is a group achievement share it – *Thanks everyone, that was a job well done.*

Recognizing and drawing satisfaction from the goals we achieve motivates us towards those goals we are still working on. Many of the children I foster have very low self-esteem, feeling they are worthless and haven't achieved anything, simply because no one has praised them for something they have done well. Praising them for even minor achievements starts them on the road to greater self-confidence so that they feel able to tackle bigger tasks. They develop and grow.

Every one of us can achieve on a daily basis, even if what we achieve is something relatively small or mundane, for example fixing the latch on the side gate or tackling the week's ironing. By accomplishing a goal we draw strength from its achievement, no matter how big or small.

Some people are very good at setting goals, short- and long-term, and do so automatically, without much conscious thought. They spring out of bed each morning, focused, with a clear idea of what they are aiming for that day, week, month or year, or in five years' time. This is fantastic, although if you are one of these people you need to make sure your dedication and focus doesn't exclude the here and now. It is essential to live in and enjoy the present while you strive for and achieve your goals; otherwise you will wake up in middle age, accomplished, successful, financially secure but wondering where life went. Goals should be balanced: have your sights set on what you want to achieve but also take pleasure in what is going on around you in the here and now.

How to set and achieve goals

For those who haven't yet developed the habit of automatically setting and achieving goals, the technique can be easily learnt. The following is a straightforward and simple practice to train your mind to set goals, and it works very well.

1. Focus on the next day. At night, as you relax in bed, before you go to sleep, spend a few moments focusing on the following day. Not to the extent of stressing yourself and keeping yourself awake but viewing the day as if watching it on television, like a soap if you wish.

2. Briefly run through what you have planned for the following day and the outcomes you are hoping for: i.e. your short-term goals. Even though much of the day is likely to be routine, it will still contain goals.

Let's say you are home based, raising your children. You will be aiming to get yourself and the children up and dressed, have breakfast, maybe with a school or nursery run, followed by shopping and housework, with a break when you hope to finish the novel you have been reading. Your aim (i.e. your goal) is to do all this, to the best of your ability, calmly and in good time. You might factor in an additional goal of joining a mothers and toddlers group to meet other mothers, or brushing up on your IT skills for when you return to work. Or maybe you will set yourself an altruistic goal of going to visit the elderly lady down the road with a bunch of flowers. All these are short-term goals and when treated as such give your life added meaning, and therefore happiness and contentment.

If you go out to work, to remind yourself of your short-term goals you might say to yourself: *Tomorrow I need to write the report for Tuesday's meeting, and phone Brian to see if he wants to play squash after work.*

If your short-term goal is part of a long-term goal, as keeping your IT skills going is in the first example, then acknowledge the long-term goal it is part of: this will keep you focused and motivated towards the aimed-for achievement.

3. Remind yourself of your goals first thing in the morning, as you shower and dress and fire up for the day ahead.

These small 'snapshots' of the day ahead are invaluable for defining and focusing on goals, and therefore make achieving them more likely.

4. At the end of the day acknowledge the achievement of your goals, no matter how small they seem, and enjoy the satisfaction that comes with it. Even if nothing out of the ordinary happened, still acknowledge your achievement and congratulate yourself. For example: *I got the kids to school on time, cleaned the house and typed that letter of complaint.*

5. Turn any unfinished tasks into new goals. If there were tasks you didn't complete in the day and have to return to, carry them over to the next day. In this way they become new goals. Congratulating yourself on what you did achieve and setting what you didn't as a new goal is a way of thinking and acting positively that means you don't beat yourself up when you fall short of your aim but instead focus on what you did well and how best to complete the tasks.

6. Make a list. If you are likely to forget your goals, short- or long-term, then write them down. I am a great believer in notelets. I couldn't get by without them, and these are in addition to my diary and work plan for writing. Make a list of your goals like a shopping list, and tick them off as you achieve them.

A list for one day for me might look something like this:

Take Alex to contact, 9.30
Buy paint for bedroom
Edit article for website
Shop – bread, cheese, fruit
Collect Alex 12.30
Draft outline of chapter two while Alex has his nap
Dinner – fish?
Watch holiday programme on Egypt 8.00 p.m. Next
   year's holiday?

This list contains some short-term goals – for example, taking Alex to contact and shopping – while others are part of longer-term goals – drafting the outline of chapter two for a book that will take a year to write and watching the television programme for a possible holiday next year. Although some of these goals could be described as routine or mundane, they are no less important and if I strive to achieve them to the best of my ability I will take pleasure in having done them.

Writing down your goals and ticking them off has the added bonus of allowing you to see exactly how much you achieve in a day. While it might be a reality check for some (who perhaps need to set and achieve more goals), for many it comes as a pleasant surprise to see how much we do achieve in an average day.

Vision

We all have at least one vision which is personal to us. We could call it our ultimate dream. It is that hope, that aspiration, that longed-for achievement that we work towards and will never give up on even if it takes a lifetime to accomplish. Often we don't tell anyone about our vision, or possibly we share it only with our closest loved ones, until we are close to achieving it or have achieved it. As I mentioned earlier, we may also have a vision on a global level, such as enough food and clean water for all, world peace, and end to cruelty and abuse. We do what we can to achieve our global vision by donating to charities, signing petitions, demonstrating and voting, etc, but largely we have to leave our global vision in the hands of our country's elected leaders, frustrating though this can be at times.

Fortunately, however, our personal vision – and how it can be attained – is safely in our own hands and therefore achievable. It may have a dream-like quality and it may sometimes appear to be outside our reach, but it will be something we can work towards. Attaining our vision is not easy; many visions are ones that take a lifetime to achieve. But the happiness and sense of fulfilment once we have our dream is like no other. All the years of hard work are worthwhile.

I spent thirty years with the vision that one day I would have a book published. I was writing short stories, articles, etc., but like so many aspiring writers the book deal kept escaping me. My vision wasn't for material gain but for the recognition of me as a writer – that a publisher liked my book enough to want to publish it. It was a stamp of approval. Thirty years is a long time to nurture and work towards a vision, but although my confidence took quite a few knocks I never gave up. When I finally achieved my dream I was obviously ecstatic, as was my family, with whom I finally shared my dream on the day the book arrived in the shops.

If I hadn't attained my vision would I have continued working towards it? Undoubtedly. Although we might have to adapt our vision, we never give up on it. I know a man who is seventy-five and is about to fulfil his lifetime dream of sailing around the world. He says he's had to accept that it would be unwise to attempt the voyage single-handed now, as he'd hoped to do as a younger man, but nevertheless he will achieve his vision by being part of a crew.

Our personal vision doesn't have to be 'sensible'; in fact it often isn't. Very few of our dreams are based on common sense and practicality. But our vision does have to be attainable. It is no use having a vision of wanting to be a famous singer if you can't sing – as many *X Factor* contestants have found out to their great distress. Or becoming a famous footballer if you never learn to play football. Visions can be fantastical but not fanciful; if they are fanciful we set ourselves up for frustration, disappointment and failure.

My guess is that as you are reading this you have a warm frisson of recognition. Maybe your vision is to travel to the Far East, work in an orphanage, climb Everest, scuba dive, parachute, paint pictures, own your own company or, like me, write books. Your vision is more elaborate and far-reaching than your long-term goal but it is important to you and you owe it to yourself to nurture it alongside your daily life until it reaches fruition, when you can quietly glow in your achievement. And if someone shares their vision with you, consider yourself very privileged and give them all the encouragement they need to accomplish it. Forty-five years ago Martin Luther King had a vision and its legacy is still with us today.

CHAPTER SEVEN

Look after Your Body

I never considered myself unhealthy until I got healthy. I stopped eating a lot of rubbish and started cooking myself proper meals (like my mum made). I feel so much better now – more alive, and my grades have improved. I'm sure all that junk food was affecting my brain. Some days it was all I could do to stay awake. So wrote one university student in her early twenties who, like so many of us with a hectic lifestyle, had got into the habit of eating too much processed (fast) food. Changing her diet set her on course for a healthier, happier and more successful life.

Earlier we looked at the power of the mind, and how by changing our mental outlook we can live happier and more contented lives. We acknowledged that the mind and body are interconnected, our state of mind having an effect on our physical health. Now we are going to look at the effect our bodies have on our minds. As our minds are responsible for the well-being of our bodies, so our bodies play a large part in the well-being of our minds. A healthy body is essential for a healthy, happy mind, and will support you as you make changes towards leading a more positive and happier life.

A healthy body depends largely on three main factors, diet, sleep and exercise. All of these are within our control, so achieving optimum physical health – and therefore optimum mental health – is far easier than many of us imagine.

Diet

. . . .

We are what we eat. This well-known concept first appeared in 1826, when a French philosopher said, *Tell me what you eat and I will tell you what you are*, meaning that the food we eat has a bearing on our state of mind and health. In 1863 another French philosopher took the phrase a step further and declared, *A man is what he eats* ('man' being used here to denote mankind and not just males). Then in 1942 Victor Lindlahr, a nutritionist wrote a book called *You Are What You Eat*, and the idea that what we eat directly affects our state of mind as well as our bodies has gone from strength to strength, as scientific research has shown that to be so.

When we eat any food or take in fluid, levels of chemicals present in the brain – namely serotonin, endorphins and dopamine – change. These powerful chemicals affect mood, and certain foods affect the levels of these chemicals and therefore our mood. Sugar, for example, dramatically increases serotonin, a chemical that gives us a sense of feeling good. So the 'lift' we get from eating something sweet isn't a notion but a real change in the brain. Serotonin is used in some antidepressants, for example Prozac, to help stabilize a person's mood where the natural levels of serotonin are low.

Diet can help enormously in maintaining a good balance of not only serotonin but also the many other chemicals that are found in the human body. We all know that a well-balanced diet is essential to remain healthy: proteins, for instance (found in meat, eggs, fish, nuts, seeds and dairy products), are necessary for repair and healing, fighting disease and growth in children; deficiencies in vitamins and minerals cause physical problems. What many of us may not know is the importance of minerals and vitamins for our emotional health. This is an area still being researched, but the findings so far underline just how important a good diet is for our mental well-being.

Zinc, found in meat, shellfish, milk, cheese, bread and cereal, is essential for good brain functioning. A deficiency can result in mood swings, poor memory, increased emotionality and heightened levels of stress.

Magnesium, found in bread, fish, meat, dairy products, green leafy vegetables, nuts and pulses, has been described as a natural tranquilliser. A deficiency can result in restlessness and poor concentration.

B vitamins, found in meat, bread, cereals, rice, eggs, vegetables, soya beans, nuts, potatoes, dairy products, cod and salmon, are essential for the brain and nervous system to function properly. Deficiency can result in poor learning and memory, aggression and depression.

Iron, found in red meat, beans, nuts, dried fruit, brown rice, soya, dark green vegetables, fortified breakfast cereal and chocolate, is responsible for carrying oxygen around the body. A deficiency is known as anaemia and results in mental and physical exhaustion, poor attention, and low learning and work performance levels.

Omega-3 oils are found in oily fish – tuna, salmon, trout, herring, mackerel, and sardines – and can also be taken as a supplement. Omega-3 is responsible for normal development and brain functioning. A deficiency has been linked to poor memory and concentration, mood swings, depression, aggression and hyperactivity (in adults as well as children).

Fresh food is the best source for obtaining essential minerals and vitamins, as at each stage of processing food loses its natural mineral and vitamin content. Some of these minerals and vitamins are added back in later in the food processing – for example, iron and B vitamins in bread and cereal – but there is no substitute for the real thing. Don't think I am suggesting we never eat processed food; most of our lifestyles dictate we need convenience foods sometimes, and they often taste very nice. But our intake of processed food needs to be balanced with plenty of fresh food. So chicken nuggets, for example, could be served with potatoes, peas and salad; or a take-away one night could be balanced the following morning with a breakfast of fresh fruit, wholemeal toast and muesli. I love chocolate and certainly wouldn't give it up. 'Treats' are good for us, in moderation.

In extreme cases of vitamin or mineral deficiency a supplement can be prescribed, but this should only be taken on the advice of a doctor, as overdosing on vitamins and minerals can be harmful. Scientists have found that vitamins and minerals become toxic at high levels. This is particularly true of vitamins A, D, E and K, and iron, as the body has difficulty getting rid of any excess.

So while our diet should include foods that have a positive influence on our mental well-being, it is important that we have them in the right amounts. A healthy body equals a healthy mind. Now a few words of warning about some of the food and drinks that many of us love but need to keep a check on:

Sugar

For most of us eating something sweet is pleasant, and sugar in moderation is not harmful; indeed we need some sugar (preferably from fruit rather than biscuits, cake, etc.) as part of a well-balanced diet. However, in most of the developed world people eat far too many sugary foods and our sugar intake has risen dramatically in a generation. Apart from the obvious sugar-heavy foods (sweets, biscuits, cakes, etc.), sugar is regularly added to many processed foods including some bread, tinned vegetables, beans, sauces and cereals. As well as being responsible for tooth decay, obesity, diabetes and high blood pressure, there is growing evidence that too much sugar can affect our mental health.

We are all familiar with the 'sugar rush' – that immediate (but short-lived) boost of energy we experience after eating sugar-laden food. Studies have shown that this sugar 'high' can also produce panic attacks, and people who are prone to anxiety can experience an increased level of anxiety after a sugar rush, which stays high for up to five hours after the food has been eaten. While not everyone will experience anxiety or panic attacks from ingesting a sugar-laden food or drink, many of us will be very familiar with the 'low' that follows the sugar 'high' and makes us moody, irritable, lethargic and short on patience and concentration, as our blood-sugar level, and therefore our energy level, falls as quickly as it rose. The energy boost from sugar is very short and sugar can be addictive. So when you crave instant energy, instead of reaching for a chocolate bar you would do better eating a banana, which provides three natural sugars – sucrose, fructose and glucose – and starch for instant and sustained energy; or a cheese sandwich, which dispenses its energy slowly over a longer period.

Caffeine

Caffeine is the most widely used mood-altering drug in the world, and it is legal. Caffeine, found in coffee, is a powerful stimulant and over 80 per cent of adults regularly drink coffee, and tea (which also contains some caffeine). In moderation caffeine it is not harmful and its effects are positive, making us alert and sociable, with increased energy and feelings of happiness and well-being. However, regular large doses of caffeine can make us anxious, nervous and agitated, and give us the physical side effects of heart palpitations, raised blood pressure and upset stomach. So if you experience any of these symptoms for no obvious reason, check your intake of caffeine.

Most of us who regularly drink coffee will be mildly addicted to caffeine – the pressing need for a cup of coffee first thing in the morning is in fact the need to counteract the effect of overnight withdrawal. Mild addiction isn't a problem, but problems can arise as a result of caffeine being added to many fizzy drinks, so that our addiction is far greater than we realize, and we don't associate the symptoms we experience with caffeine withdrawal. I have come across children as young as six and seven who were addicted to caffeine because of their high consumption of fizzy drinks. Even slight withdrawal can include headaches, fatigue, drowsiness, difficulty concentrating, irritability, depression, anxiety and flu-like symptoms. If you experience any of these symptoms for no obvious reason, again check your level of caffeine intake and if necessary reduce your consumption. Being addicted to anything – even sugar or caffeine – will not promote a positive mindset.

Alcohol

Many cultures view drinking alcohol in moderation as socially acceptable, and in moderation alcohol consumption is not detrimental to our long-term health; indeed some studies suggest the occasional drink is good for us. However, there is growing concern in many countries at the increased levels of alcohol consumption, which are causing physical and metal health problems on an unprecedented scale, even in teenagers. Alcohol, while pleasant and not harmful in small quantities, becomes poisonous at high levels, and our bodies (especially our livers) have to work very hard to get rid of the toxins.

When we have an alcoholic drink, initially we feel more relaxed and sociable, and inhibitions can vanish as the alcohol reaches the cognitive areas of the brain. Physically, our heart rates speed up slightly, giving us a warm glow as small blood vessels dilate and more blood flows to the surface of the skin. But alcohol is a depressant, not a stimulant, so very soon we start to lose the 'feel-good effect' alcohol produces unless we have another drink. Drinking to excess is very dangerous, resulting in vomiting, liver damage, memory loss, unconsciousness, coma and even death. Even moderate regular drinking can result in increased anxiety, depression, mood swings, irritability and sleeping problems. Alcohol is present in two-thirds of suicide attempts, and 50 per cent of alcoholics suffer from a mental illness. Alcohol dependency changes the way the brain works and can result in hallucinations, psychosis, obsessive compulsive behaviour and paranoia.

People vary in their tolerance to alcohol: some people are less adept at processing out the toxins than others. These people are more susceptible to the harmful effects of alcohol, and it will damage their bodies faster. Women have less tolerance to alcohol than men, and as we get older our tolerance diminishes. Children have no tolerance of alcohol and should never be given it. Guidelines to safe drinking have been issued in many countries, so if you drink alcohol, check you are within the guidelines, and that you are in control of your drinking. If you find you *need* a drink and search out alcohol, then the chances are you're not in control and alcohol is in control of you.

This was the case for one successful businessman in his mid-thirties, who wrote: *Many of our contracts were won over a long lunch with plenty of wine; then I'd often stop off for a drink after work, and meet the lads for a drink at weekends. I drank, but no more than anyone else. I never considered I had a drink problem. Then I had a medical for work and it showed I had liver damage. I was horrified. I'd had no symptoms. I've been off the booze for two years now and I feel so much better, not only physically but mentally. I still go for the lunches but have fruit juice instead. It's weird watching others become intoxicated: the more they drink the less sense they make.*

And a woman in her late twenties who was feeling isolated, having given up work to look after her children, thought she could find comfort in a bottle. She wrote: *The glass of wine with my lunch became two, then three, so that by the time my partner came home from work I'd drunk a bottle and was opening the next. This went on every day for over a year. I was so tired and hung over I was barely functioning. I also got very depressed. I'm sure it was the booze – I'd never suffered from depression before. I never felt fully awake or capable of doing anything well. My confidence was nil. It was my partner who finally brought it to a head. We had a blazing row and he said I wasn't fit to look after the children. He was right. It was the wake-up call I needed. I shudder to think I was in charge of the children while drunk. Now I only have a drink with others when we go out or have a dinner party. As soon as I stopped drinking the depression lifted. I feel like I've been given a second chance, and I'm making it up to my children.*

Happiness and contentment do not come in a bottle; indeed alcohol abuse (of which the two cases above are examples) will hinder you from adopting a positive mindset and stop you achieving your goals. Regular heavy drinking will damage you physically and mentally, over a relatively short period – months not years. If you are not drinking alcohol within the safety guidelines and need to reduce your intake, but can't do so alone, seek help from your doctor or a support group.

Food containing additives

Although much has been written about the effects of certain food additives (known as E numbers) on children, not so much has been documented about the effect additives have on adults. Food additives are added to food processing for reasons of appearance, shelf life, texture and taste. All additives have to be tested and pass food safety standards, but research studies have shown some E numbers can cause unpleasant side effects and even illness in some of the population. People vary in their tolerance to additives and most people will have no adverse reaction to them, but if you have unexplained symptoms it might be worth looking on the packet or tin of any processed foods you have been eating to see what has been added, and consider the following:

Monosodium glutamate (E621), usually used as a flavour enhancer, can cause palpitations, sleeplessness, behavioural reactions, headaches, dizziness, chest pains, depression and mood swings. Found in many processed foods including soups and ready-made meals.

Preservatives (BHA, BHT, EDTA, etc.) can aggravate Attention Deficit and Hyperactivity Disorder (ADD and ADHD) and trigger poor concentration and restlessness. Used instead of the traditional preservatives of salt, vinegar and oil, preservatives are found in many processed foods.

Sunset yellow (E110) can cause or aggravate hyperactivity, poor concentration and memory retention. Found in orange squash, orange jelly, marzipan, Swiss roll, apricot jam, citrus marmalade, lemon curd, sweets, hot chocolate mix, packet soups, breadcrumbs, cheese sauce, ice cream, canned fish and many medications. Allowed in the UK, but banned in Norway and Finland.

Quinoline yellow (E104) has been linked to ADHD, restlessness and irritability. Found in ices, Scotch eggs, smoked haddock, hair products, colognes and a wide range of medications. Allowed in the UK, but banned in Australia, Japan, Norway and the United States.

Carmoisine (E122) has been linked to ADHD, sleeplessness and loss of concentration. Found in blancmange, marzipan, Swiss roll, jams and preserves, sweets, brown sauce, flavoured yoghurts, packet soups, jellies, breadcrumbs and cheesecake mixes. Allowed in the UK, but banned in Japan, Norway, Sweden and the United States.

Allura red (E129) can cause or aggravate ADHD and is linked to irritability and lack of concentration. Found in sweets, drinks, sauces, medications and cosmetics. Not allowed in food and drink for children under three. Banned in Denmark, Belgium, France, Germany, Switzerland, Sweden, Austria and Norway.

Tartrazine (E102): many people are allergic to it and it has been shown to cause and aggravate ADHD. Found in fruit squash, fruit cordial, coloured fizzy drinks, instant puddings, cake mixes, custard powder, soups, sauces, ice cream, ice lollies, sweets, chewing gum, marzipan, jam, jelly, marmalade, mustard, yoghurt and many convenience foods. Widely used in the UK, but banned in Norway and Austria.

Ponceau 4R (E124) is linked to ADHD and sleep disturbance. Found in dessert toppings, jelly, salami, seafood dressings, tinned strawberries, fruit pie fillings, cake mixes, cheesecakes, soups and trifles. Allowed in the UK, but banned in Norway and the United States.

Additives only appear in processed food, which is another reason for eating as much fresh and unprocessed food as possible. For while not everyone will suffer adverse reactions ingesting these additives, they certainly won't do you any good.

Water

Water is largely free and available and you should drink plenty of it. Two-thirds of our body weight is water; 80 per cent of the human brain is water; 82 per cent of our blood is water; and 90 per cent of our lungs is water. Water is crucial to our physical and mental health. A drop of 2 per cent in the body's water can result in dehydration, resulting in fatigue, problems concentrating, poor short-term memory and trouble focusing. By the time you feel thirsty you are already dehydrated, and even mild dehydration can cause headaches, tiredness, loss of concentration and irritability. Salt, which is added to many snacks and processed food, is a diuretic – i.e. it makes you wee more, which results in dehydration if the lost fluid is not replaced.

It is essential to keep our bodies and brains hydrated to function effectively and positively, so drink regularly. It doesn't have to be plain water: tea and coffee (in moderation), fruit juice and squashes are all water based and count towards your fluid intake.

Sleep

Sufficient sleep, too, is vital for physical health and for maintaining a positive, healthy outlook on life. The exact amount of sleep adults need varies from person to person, but it is generally accepted that six to eight hours of uninterrupted sleep a night is ideal. Babies, young children and pregnant women need more sleep, while the elderly need less. When we sleep we heal, physically and mentally.

Sleep performs a number of essential functions. While we sleep our bodies fight infection – which is why we take to our beds and sleep more when we are ill. Babies, children and young adults grow in their sleep. No, it's not a myth: growth hormones are released in sleep. Sleep also allows us to dream, and dreaming is vital for a healthy mind. It allows our fears and anxieties, buried deep in the subconscious, to surface in an acceptable form, so that we deal with them. Studies have shown that having enough dream sleep (REM) is as important, if not more important, than having enough sleep. Some medications, including antidepressants and sleeping pills, inhibit REM, as does evening alcohol consumption.

We can't live without sleep. While there have been no studies of extreme sleep deprivation on humans (for obvious reasons), in a study of rats, who normally have a lifespan of between two and three years, the rats died after three weeks when deprived of sleep. Sleep deprivation is a recognized form of torture, which, to the human race's shame, is sometimes used as a means of interrogating prisoners of war; apparently it is very effective. Even short-term sleep deprivation can result in poor concentration and memory recall, irritability, irrational anxieties and a reduced ability to cope with minor crisis. The effect of sleep deprivation is cumulative, and not getting enough sleep over a long period can lead to depression, acute anxiety, hallucinations and even psychosis.

We all suffer from lack of sleep sometimes – because of a late-night party, a new baby, noisy neighbours, worrying about something – and we usually make up the lost sleep as best we can in the following days. If you find yourself awake in the middle of the night, worrying about a seemingly unfathomable problem, don't. Tell yourself you will deal with it the following morning and then concentrate on going back to sleep. Many books and websites detail techniques for getting back to sleep which focus on relaxing the body and mind – everything from counting sheep to self-hypnosis. If I wake in the early hours worrying about something, I find listening to the radio (without the light on) helps, as my thoughts fix on what is being said rather than the overload of information buzzing around my head. However, if you suffer from chronic insomnia, then you should seek medical help.

Establishing a soothing bedtime routine that relaxes you physically and mentally helps pave the way for a good night's sleep. This might include a bath, a warm drink or making love. Avoid working late, studying or surfing the net immediately before bed, as these increase brain activity at a time when you should be reducing it in preparation for sleep. Fortunately for most people, not getting enough sleep is a result of their lifestyle and therefore within their control, rather than acute insomnia: that is, a lot of people simply go to bed too late, even when they have to get up at a set time in the morning. If you're one of them, don't. Whether you are running the country, a large corporation or your home, whether you are studying or job seeking, it is essential to have enough sleep to stay healthy physically and mentally and reach your full potential.

Exercise

● ●

You don't have to go to the gym each day or jog for miles around the streets, unless you want to of course. Walking instead of using the car (if practical), or taking the steps rather than the lift, is good exercise as it stimulates the heart and circulatory system. If you incorporate exercise into your daily routine rather than going out of your way to achieve it, you are far more likely to continue with it. How many of us have taken up gym membership with very good intentions only to find that going to the gym two or three times a week really didn't fit in with our lifestyle? So walking (briskly, not dawdling), housework, gardening and washing the car are all forms of exercise and have the added advantage of achieving more than just fitness – money saved on petrol, pollution reduced, a clean house or car, a tidy garden, etc.

Most of us will be aware of the benefits to our physical health of exercise, which include reduced risk of heart disease, high blood pressure, stroke, diabetes, obesity, osteoporosis and even cancer. Not so many of us will be aware of the positive effect exercise has on our minds. So convincing is the evidence for this that doctors now regularly prescribe exercise when treating depression and other mental illnesses. Not only has exercise been shown to relieve depression, anxiety and stress but it can also reduce the likelihood of succumbing to another bout of depression, anxiety or stress, as well as raising our self-esteem, motivation and concentration.

Why?

When we exercise, our levels of serotonin and endorphins go up (just as they do when we smile or eat sweet food). I have already mentioned that these natural chemicals, released by the brain, are responsible for mood, and raised levels make us feel good. In fact, the feel-good effect of exercise can be so great that athletes or those who train hard can become addicted to the 'high' exercise creates. Research evidence has proved the work these endorphins do. In experiments when endorphins were injected into depressed patients their mood improved.

How exercise encourages a positive mind

Physical exercise has also been shown to encourage a healthy and positive mind by:

1. Giving us a sense of purpose – a goal or positive focus, whether it is lifting a certain level of weights at the gym, swimming a set number of lengths or achieving a clean car or a tidy house and garden.

2. Boosting our self-esteem so that we feel good about ourselves and the way we look.

3. Making us feel less isolated by encouraging us to meet people. Joining a badminton or tennis club, for example, will increase your circle of friends. I know if I am at home and want a chat I go into my front garden with a pair of secateurs and begin snipping the shrubs, and it won't be long before a passerby or someone I know stops for a chat. Likewise washing the car outside the house often attracts neighbours with a friendly call of *You can do mine next!*

A survey by MIND (a charity for mental health) found that an amazing 83 per cent of people with mental health problems used physical exercise to make them feel better. What better testament could there be to the positive power of exercise to help us achieve a happy and contented life.

CHAPTER EIGHT

Be Body Positive

In Chapters Three and Four we saw how important it is to act positively as well as think positively if we are to achieve happiness and contentment. Now we are going to take 'act positively' a stage further and address the importance of developing a **positive body image.** Quite simply, if we are to feel good on the inside we need to look good on the outside too.

This is not about trying to conform to some unrealistic media image of a model of perfection (responsible for so much frustration and sadness, especially in women). It is about achieving our personal best. Being body positive is about making the very best of what you have and making your appearance work for you so that you feel good.

Appearance is important, although some might try to tell us otherwise. Our appearance is usually the first aspect of us another person encounters. Rightly or wrongly, we make many assumptions about a person based on that first sighting. Research has shown that our initial impression of someone is very difficult to change afterwards, even when subsequent encounters suggest differently. In the first few seconds of meeting someone new we judge a person on many attributes, including their honesty, likeability, integrity, confidence and reliability, basing our judgement solely on what we see. And amazingly, research has shown that our first impression is accurate. In one piece of research subjects were shown 20–30-second video clips of job applicants greeting their interviewers, and were asked to rank the applicants' characteristics – honesty, integrity, self-assurance, etc. Their assessments were shown to be as reliable as those of the professionally trained interviewers who spent at least twenty minutes interviewing each applicant.

It is thought our ability to make a snapshot valid judgement when we meet someone for the first time developed with our early ancestors in a primitive part of the brain. Their lives would have depended on making a quick decision on whether someone was going to help or harm them and whether they needed to run.

A blind person uses other senses – smell, touch and hearing – to create a mental picture of a person they are meeting for the first time. They will also make assumptions about that person based on the 'visual' image they create, which will subsequently be difficult to shake.

Not only is our appearance crucial to how other people perceive us but it is also a good indicator of how we perceive ourselves. Our appearance tells those we come in contact with how we see ourselves, how we rank ourselves and in effect how we are feeling at any given moment. If we are feeling good about ourselves the other person is likely to feel good about us too.

It is, therefore, essential that our appearance sends the message that we are positive, happy, self-assured and at one with the world, not only for the benefit of others but also for ourselves. Research has also shown that if we are feeling a bit down, then upping our appearance, for example by wearing something new or visiting the hairdresser, will make us feel better on the inside too.

Our body image comprises a number of areas that go to make up our appearance – that is, our outer self. Let us look at each of these in turn.

Body language

There has been much research on the subject of body language, and there are books and websites dedicated to helping us interpret each other's body language. Briefly, body language is the manner in which we move, stand, sit, greet and leave people, and generally hold ourselves and what that communicates to others. Our body language gives off lots of subtle signs about how we feel about ourselves, which those we meet subconsciously note and interpret. We therefore need to express ourselves positively through our body language and this is how:

1. When standing, stand upright with your head held high. To achieve this, draw back your shoulders and take a deep breath. If you can't take a deep breath then you are not standing upright (our lungs deflate when we slouch, reducing our intake of oxygen). Stand with your feet slightly apart: this suggests self-confidence and that you are open to interaction.

2. When walking, hold yourself upright, with your arms loosely at your sides, and walk with purpose. This reflects the fact that you are a positive person who has many aims in life.

3. When you sit, keep your back upright and supported against the chair, unless of course you're relaxing on the sofa or propped on the bed.

4. Don't fiddle – with your tie, necklace, hair, teeth, fingers, cuff, etc. As well as making others nervous it suggests you are nervous, or bored with their company, and that you may be unreliable, with something to hide. Keep your hands inactive, loosely folded in your lap or hanging at your sides, unless they are gainfully employed, for example in writing. It is fine to gesticulate to emphasize a point but don't overdo it: it's distracting.

5. Make eye contact. This reflects confidence, openness, co-operation and honesty. But don't stare: it makes others uncomfortable. In conversation it's acceptable to glance away every ten seconds or so (we usually do this automatically).

6. Remember to smile. Smiling is the most positive and welcoming signal you can give. It will tell everyone you are happy, good natured, approachable, warm, friendly and comfortable with yourself.

Clothes

• •

In my role as a foster carer I was recently interviewed for an article to be published in a magazine circulated to social workers. One of the questions was: *If you were the director of children's services, what changes would you make to the system?* Plenty! I gave a number of heartfelt and well-considered suggestions for making improvements in the child protection system so that we can better safeguard our children and stop abuse. I ended on a lighter note with: *Educate social workers (particularly men) on basic dress code. It is not OK to arrive at a meeting in washed-out jeans, open-toed sandals and a creased shirt, looking as though they've just fallen out of bed.* It was a light-hearted jibe at how some social workers dress, but I meant it. I've sat in meetings and been appalled at what some social workers think is acceptable dress for a formal meeting. Clothes don't just give us warmth and protection but make a statement about our values, personalities and role, how we expect to be treated and the importance we place on the occasion. Which in this example of the meeting clearly wasn't much. We are judged by our clothes. They give off silent messages just as our body language does, and others will pick up these messages and make assumptions about you based on them. To be perceived as a successful and whole rounded person you need to dress appropriately.

The clothes you wear in your leisure time will largely be your choice, but your choice of clothes for work will have to conform to certain norms if you are to be taken as serious and competent in your role. However, within these norms there is room for personal choice. If you are uncertain what is appropriate wear for work, look around your workplace and see what others are wearing. If you are still uncertain ask your boss.

The following example, possibly extreme, demonstrates the power of clothing. A man who worked in a large fashionable department store was undergoing hormone treatment in preparation for a sex change operation so that he could live his life as a woman. He had been wearing men's clothing for work but his psychologist said that he now needed to start dressing as a woman all the time in the last stage before he went ahead with the operation that would change his gender for good. Unsure how the company would react if he suddenly arrived in women's clothes, he explained his situation to management, who were already aware of the treatment he was having. They were sympathetic and advised staff to be understanding. The following day when the man arrived in women's clothes there were a few comments, mainly positive, and by the end of the week it was no longer a topic of conversation. In the eyes of his colleagues, and the public whom he served, he was now a woman and was treated as such, so powerful is the image our clothes portray.

Clothes should be clean with no frayed edges or loose buttons – stained, worn or untidy clothes send very negative messages. They need to fit – clothes that are too tight will make you feel big and ungainly as well as looking unsightly. They should feel comfortable and sit lightly on the skin; don't wear clothes that chafe or irritate because that's exactly how you will feel: chafed and irritated.

Not only do clothes make a powerful statement about the person we are or the work we do, but they can have a direct effect on our mood and personality. If you are wearing jeans and T-shirt, for example, you are more likely to be relaxed and impulsive than if you are wearing a suit. If you are looking good, you will feel good too.

The **colour** of the clothes we wear also sends messages which reflect and can even change our mood:

* **Black:** powerful and authoritative
* **White:** innocent and pure
* **Red:** feisty, emotional and intense
* **Pink:** calm
* **Blue:** tranquil and loyal
* **Green:** relaxed
* **Dark Green:** conservative

* **Yellow:** optimistic
* **Purple:** sophisticated.

You will probably find you automatically chose the colour that best reflects your mood but if you use colour to change your mood (as research has shown that you can) you will have to consciously wear a different colour.

General presentation

Being body positive includes every aspect of how you present yourself: skin care, for instance, for both men and women. We obviously know the importance of keeping the skin clean by showering and washing regularly, but so many of us skip moisturizing. Don't! If your skin feels good, then you will feel good in your skin.

Hair is possibly our single most important feature, which is why in television makeovers the new hairstyle is only revealed, as a finale, at the end. A new hairstyle can transform a person in appearance and also make them feel more vivacious and confident.

While culture, fashion and personal taste vary and the details of how you present yourself will be a matter of individual judgement and circumstance, when considering the details of your appearance ask yourself the following:

1. Is it appropriate? As well as clothing, hairstyle (colour and length) needs to be appropriate for the occasion, whether it's work or leisure. So a purple Mohican is fine if you are a DJ on a radio show, but not if you are a high court judge. With body hair, piercings and tattoos, make sure that they are acceptable in the society in which you live and that they don't count against you.

2. Is it complementary? We are all beautiful, and being body positive is about making the best of what we have. Does your make-up, if you wear any, enhance your natural beauty rather than obliterate it? Does your hairstyle complement your features and make the statement you want it to? Hair can say much about you as a person: short hair (practical, honest and direct); long flowing hair (sensual, approachable, sexy, impulsive); thick and shining (healthy); long hair tied back (organized and business-like); chin length with a fringe (trustworthy and dependable) – note how many women politicians adopt this last style.

3. Is it comfortable? Shoes that fit properly (ladies, with heels that you can walk in); hair that is manageable; and clothes that are comfortable as well as attractive will make you feel better.

4. Is it positive? Not taking care with your appearance suggests laziness on your part and sends a negative message to others which in turn has a negative effect on you. Conversely making the most of your appearance portrays a person with high self-esteem, so others will treat you with the respect you deserve. Clothes don't have to be expensive or brand new, just clean and worn with dignity. And knowing you are looking good will lift your spirits even on a dark day.

Weight

• •

Size does matter when it comes to your body image, especially in European culture. I am not talking here about trying to emulate the undernourished models of the catwalks or fashion magazines, but about being a sensible weight, which is important for your health and body image. Rightly or wrongly you will be judged on your size. Just as someone who is badly underweight will be deemed to be ill or have eating problems (and therefore psychological problems), so being badly overweight will give out the message you are out of control of your eating and therefore your life. Other assumptions made about the obese is that they are lazy, stupid, greedy and selfish. I fully appreciate this is not true of large people but that is how many will perceive and treat you, and that will undermine your confidence and well being. Find a weight that suits you and stay with it. I have been 8½ stone all my life, except when I was pregnant. A stable and healthy weight is essential for your physical health as it is for maintaining happiness and contentment.

CHAPTER NINE

Be an Optimist

An optimist is a person who anticipates the best possible outcome for a situation, even if the odds are stacked against them. Optimists believe that people and events are generally good, and most situations work out for the best in the end. In Chapter Three I used the maxim that an optimist sees the glass half full (rather than half empty). **Optimism and positive thought go hand in hand**, so that as you train your mind to think positively you will be training your outlook to be one of optimism.

The opposite of an optimist is a pessimist, a person who anticipates the worst outcome for any given situation, even when the odds of a good outcome are overwhelmingly in their favour. However, sometimes we need a little pessimism to give us a reality check or keep us safe and not taken advantage of. This type of pessimism is better described as scepticism, which in moderation is healthy and necessary and part of everyone's life. The following statements are examples of healthy scepticism:

We've only been dating two weeks. I think it's too soon for her to be telling me she loves me; she doesn't know me yet.

I'm going to do my best at the interview but I realize I may not be offered the job; the other candidates have far more experience than me.

Why is this man emailing and asking me to invest in his business if it is making him so much money?

All the above statements have an element of pessimism but in the acceptable form of healthy scepticism. Each person is raising a sensible doubt which helps them to protect themselves. In the first example the man is right to be hesitant about his new girlfriend's protestations of love after dating for only two weeks: she should take time to get to know him. In example two the person going for a job interview rightly cautions himself about the competition he will be up against while retaining his positive outlook that he will do his best, so that he won't be disproportionately disappointed. Example three is something all those who use email will be familiar with – the scam, the investment opportunity that is too good to miss, sent from a person or company we have never heard of. People are taken in by these ruses and persuaded to part with their money when a little pessimism in the form of scepticism would have protected them.

But while it is healthy, wise and indeed sometimes essential to show some degree of pessimism and be cautious, if you are always pessimistic happiness and contentment will be very difficult to achieve. You will miss opportunities, be mistrustful of others and in effect become a 'Doubting Thomas' who believes the world and the people in it are against you and that situations always turn out for the worst:

It always happens to me!

I never win anything.

Trust no one but yourself.

You can hear the distrust and cynicism in these statements and know the person will very likely get exactly the negative outcome they envisage, so reinforcing their pessimism.

Evidence suggests those who view life optimistically are luckier, win more competitions, achieve more, are healthier and wealthier and even live longer (by 19 per cent!) than those who are cynical and pessimistic. Research is ongoing to find out why, but there appears to be a causal link between anticipating good and positive (optimism) and achieving it. Conversely, those with a pessimistic outlook achieve less, have more accidents, and are 16 per cent more likely to die during a given period compared to the average person. On all levels, therefore, we owe it to ourselves to be optimistic, guaranteeing we get the best from life, but how?

Read through the following and read it again. Then practise what you are not already doing. Changing your attitude to one of optimism will be a conscious act to begin with, but very soon you will be doing it automatically and optimism will become part of who you are.

How to be an optimist

• •

1. Understand the world is not against you. There is no unseen plot that puts obstacles in your way. You have the same opportunity as everyone else to achieve and be happy.

2. Embrace the new. Don't shy away from opportunity because it involves a measured risk.

3. Bad past experience does not equal bad future experience. History will not repeat itself; just the opposite, in fact, because you will have learnt from your past mistakes and are therefore less likely to repeat them in the future.

4. You are in control of your life; life is not in control of you. Life is a fantastic journey that can take us wherever we choose.

5. Accept that you will be unhappy sometimes. You need to feel sadness to appreciate happiness.

6. Reflect on all you have to be grateful for – loved ones, a home, enough food to eat – and be grateful for all you have.

7. Always have something to look forward to, and look forward to it as a child looks forward to Christmas. This may be a family birthday, a holiday, buying a new outfit, or curling up with a good book at the end of a tiring day. It doesn't have to be a big event, but take pleasure from the anticipated joy.

8. Live your life in the here and now. Although it is good to look forward to treats, if you don't live life in the here and now, you'll miss the good and beauty which surrounds you. Take a moment to appreciate it (see Chapter Fourteen).

9. Limit bad news – from television, radio, newspapers, etc. The media is a wonderful instrument to keep us informed but it can mean we are subjected to too much news of suffering and violence over which we have no control.

10. Accept disappointment and let it fuel your drive and ambition – *I didn't get that job but I will get the next one.*

11. Always visualize the best outcome for a future event. By focusing on the positive your optimism will shine through and increase your chances of a positive outcome.

12. Encourage others to be optimistic. As well as reinforcing your own optimism it will make others happier and warm to you. No one really wants to be reminded of the worst-case scenario. We thrive on hope and encouragement and appreciate those who point it out, as long as the sentiment is sincere.

A woman, now aged twenty-three, who as a teenager had lived on the streets of London for three years wrote: *I'll never forget Martha. She was a volunteer at the drop-in centre where I used to go. She was a big woman, larger than life, who always had a good word to say about everything and everyone. No matter how bad my life got on the streets, I knew I could go into that centre and just being around her and hearing her talk was a great lift. Everyone who used to visit the centre said the same. Her favourite expression was 'I can only give you a cup of tea and my good humour, but it's free and never runs dry.'*

What a lovely sentiment! I'm sure I would have liked Martha very much. You just know she was a truly positive person, bubbling with optimism and good will.

Be Decisive

We are all faced with decisions every minute of every waking day: what to have for breakfast, what to wear, whether to take the car or walk/accept the party invitation/ ask that girl out/voice our opinion or stay quiet. Life is one long decision-making process and the results of our decisions shape our lives at home and work, as well as affecting the lives of others. Being indecisive will result in missed opportunities and feelings of frustration and negativity. It is, therefore, crucial to your happiness and contentment to be able to make considered decisions within a reasonable time.

Decisions range in their importance and complexity, but when making a decision we all use the same basic decision-making strategy. We learnt it as children and then continued to build on it into adulthood. It isn't a skill we consciously learn like the alphabet or the times tables but a mental process that develops as a result of being presented with choices and making decisions – large and small. It is worth taking a look at what exactly goes on in our brains when we make a decision:

1. We clarify and assess the issue that needs to be decided.

2. We gather the information we need to make the decision.

3. We compare the pros and cons of each option.

4. We select the best option and make the decision.

The process is the same for small or large decisions, although the timescale will vary and is usually dependent on the complexity and enormity of the decision before us. Deciding whether to accept an invitation to go out for a drink or which dress to wear are decisions that can be processed in seconds, whereas deciding whether you should relocate, for example, or if your mother should move in with you, would normally require more time. However, if you are not to miss opportunities you need to make *all* decisions within a realistic time frame, appropriate to the depth and number of options before you and the information that you need to gather. Decisions are never *not* made: even if we take the easiest option and do nothing, the decision is still made through our inaction, although the result might not be in our best interest or those affected by our decision. It is, therefore, much better to make an informed decision based on the information available; even if it turns out to be the wrong one, lessons will have been learnt. In addition, we all warm to those who are decisive, as they make us feel secure and confident in their ability to make the right decision.

People vary in their ability to make a decision but we can all learn to make better decisions in a more realistic time frame – i.e. **become more decisive.** Prolonged hesitancy and indecisiveness are almost always a result of fear (of the unknown or other's reaction) and occasionally apathy.

> Take the young man of twenty-five who knew his long-term relationship had come to an end but couldn't make the decision to tell his partner for fear of her reaction and being disliked: *I know I'm being selfish and I feel like a fraud but I stay with Sarah because it's easier. If I finish the relationship she's going to cry and be upset and all her family and friends will hate me. She keeps talking about our future together – living together and having a baby – and I sit there and nod and don't say anything. I'm sure she can't be happy with me. I guess I'm hoping that in the end she'll get fed up and finish with me. It will be so much easier.*

Yes, of course it will be easier if she finishes with him first. It would relieve him of the responsibility for the decision; of course Sarah is going to be upset when he tells her how he feels. But sometimes we need to make what seems a harsh decision at the time for the long-term benefit of not only ourselves but also those with whom we are involved. This man knew that by being indecisive as well as not being honest he was prolonging the inevitable and creating more unhappiness, when had he been decisive he and Sarah could have both been rebuilding their lives and meeting new people.

I understood from the rest of this man's letter that he was normally decisive but had (understandably) got stuck with this issue because of all the emotions involved. Some people, however, have long-term problems with decision making.

Not as unusual as you may think was the couple in America who were both indecisive. It was the woman who wrote: *I am hopeless at making decisions, and so is my husband. Even over small things. As a result we don't seem to do anything. We desperately need to move to a bigger house. We are in a two-bedroom apartment which has no garden and we have three children. We've been house hunting for five years and must have looked at over 200 properties but we can't make a decision. It's getting me down living on top of each other like this and we are all arguing. The only reason we moved into this apartment in the first place was because a friend was selling it at the time we were getting married – it was easier than house-hunting …* The woman carried on to say that she felt she and her husband were stuck in a rut because they could never make a decision to do anything different from what they had been doing since they'd first started going out at college. They hadn't been on holiday for eight years because they couldn't even make a decision where to go!

Indecision like this is based on fear of making the wrong decision. This works against us by stopping us improving our home and work lives. In the above example indecision kept the family stuck in a tiny apartment and never going on holiday (and much more) simply because the adults were frightened to make the wrong decision. *Better the devil you know* is the maxim, but it isn't true. It is far better to make an informed decision: if it is the right decision you will benefit from the results, and if it turns out to be the wrong decision you will have gained from the experience and will be better informed if you have to make a similar decision in the future.

If you are someone who often takes too long to reach a decision, or never makes an active decision, resulting in you doing nothing, it will be affecting your happiness and contentment and you need to address your indecisiveness and correct it. This is how.

How to be decisive

• •

1. Set a time limit for making the decision if there isn't one already set by external forces (for example at work). **Stick to the time limit** and don't put off until tomorrow what you can decide today.

2. Clarify the decision that needs to be made and get rid of any pre-conceived notions. So often we misinterpret a request or situation because of pre-conceived or misplaced judgemental notions.

3. Gather the information you need to make the decision.

4. Compare the pros and cons of each option.

5. Select the best option.

6. Can't select the best option? Then **address the fear** that is stopping you from making this decision. Ask yourself what it is you are afraid of. It helps to consider the negative consequences of your inaction, and the worst-case scenario if you make the wrong decision. Your fear of it won't be as bad once you have acknowledged it.

7. Make the decision and act on it.

8. Don't over-think and revisit steps three and four (which is what happens when you change your mind). You have considered all the options and made your decision. Leave it and move on.

The above schema works because it follows the way our brains work when making a decision and includes steps to get over the stumbling block of indecisiveness. These are: setting a time limit addressing your fears and not revisiting the decision once you have made it.

Perhaps you feel this is easier said than done, so let's look at how it works in practice, using the example of the couple who want to move house. When two or more are involved, the process is more complex than when only you are responsible for the decision, as others' views will have to be taken into account. But the decision-making process is the same if you are making a decision as an individual, couple, family, or large working committee in business.

1. The couple **set a time limit**, saying that by that time they will have made their decision. Given that they have already been house hunting for five years, I would suggest three months is a realistic time within which to complete their search.

2. The couple **clarify the decision** – i.e. the reasons for the decision – and they get rid of any pre-conceived notions. The reasons are that they are moving house because their present apartment is too small for their growing family. It is a practical decision for the good of the whole family. They have a pre-conceived notion that because they had problems finding somewhere suitable in the past they will do so in the future but they acknowledge that in fact that is not the case. Next they discuss and agree on the type of house they are looking for: size, number of bedrooms, location, etc.

3. The couple work together to **gather the information** they need. They register with estate agents and property-finding websites, as well as looking at the property section in the local newspaper. They make arrangements to view properties that appear to meet their criteria. After the visits they discard properties that don't meet their criteria and make a list of those that do.

4. The couple **compare the pros and cons.** They write down all the good and bad points of each property on their list.

5. They **select the best option** from the list and make an offer on the house.

6. They find they can't make the offer, so they **address the fear** that is stopping them, individually and jointly. They ask themselves what exactly are they afraid of? Losing friends? The upheaval of packing? Making the wrong choice? Then they look at the negative consequences of doing nothing: staying in an overcrowded apartment and getting on each other's nerves. They ask themselves what is the worst-case scenario if they make the wrong decision: they don't like the house/neighbours/location and have to move again. By considering all of these questions and confronting their fears the couple put their moving into a better perspective and will now feel able to make their decision.

7. They **make the decision and act on it.** That is, they make the offer on their first-choice house.

8. Having made their decision, they **don't over-think** and revisit steps three and four (so they don't change their minds). They have rationally considered all the options and have made a sensible decision based on them. If their offer isn't accepted and a deal can't be done, then they will make an offer on the next property on their list, reminding themselves of the time limit they have set for completing the task.

A word of warning: while couples can offer each other support, and share responsibility in decision making, they can also be catalysts for indecisiveness. Couples must be careful not to go down the path of feeding off each other's indecision and thereby giving it a stamp of approval, which is what must have happened to the couple in the example.

> Husband: *'Supposing the new neighbours have rowdy children or a dog that barks all night?'*

> Wife: *'I know, that's what's worrying me. At least here we know our neighbours are quiet.'*

> Husband: *'Absolutely! Better to stay put.'*

Had the wife offered a positive decisive statement in response to her husband's negative one, she would have encouraged him to think more positively:

Husband: *'Supposing the new neighbours have rowdy children or a dog that barks all night?'*

Wife: *'It's a very pleasant neighbourhood. I expect the neighbours will be nice.'*

Husband: *'Yes, and hopefully they'll have children the same age as ours so they can play together.'*

Wife: *'I love the property, it sounds fantastic!'*

Whether you are one of a couple, an individual, or part of a group or committee, practise decision-making skills at every opportunity. If you are confronted by a mammoth decision that gives you a sick feeling in the pit of your stomach then address your fear and say to yourself (or to those around you if it is a joint or group decision): 'This is a big decision, but it needs to be made as soon as possible, so let's get on with it.'

One of my father's favourite expressions when he was trying to motivate those around him to make a decision and act was: *The road to nowhere is paved with good intentions.* This is actually a misquote, a slightly watered-down version of *The road to hell is paved with good intentions* (usually attributed to Samuel Johnson, 1775). Nowhere or hell, it doesn't really matter: we all knew what my father meant: it's no use having good intentions unless you make a decision and get down to the task before you. To finish with another quote about indecisiveness made famous by the very decisive Welsh politician Aneurin Bevan (1897–1960): *We know what happens to people who stay in the middle of the road. They get run down.* So easily avoided by the decision to step out of the way.

As for the American couple in the example, they used the above decision-making strategy and are now happily settled in their new home.

....

CHAPTER ELEVEN

Use Intuition

Intuition can be described as 'quick and ready insight'. It is a way of knowing or sensing something without observation, reason or experience, sometimes called instinct or a 'gut reaction'. We have all experienced intuition at some time – about a person, a situation or a decision we were being asked to make. Intuition is usually very strong and immediate, and whether we act on it or ignore it will depend largely on the type of person we are. Creative people – musicians, writers, artists, designers, etc. – tend to be more intuitive and ready to listen to and act on their instinct, and women tend to be more intuitive than men.

Intuition often pops up when we least expect it, and research has shown that if we follow our instinct when making a decision, the decision is more than likely to turn out be the right one. This appears to fly in the face of rational and informed decision making – or does it?

Albert Einstein, generally considered to be the most accomplished scientist of the twentieth century and therefore presumably rational and level-headed, said, 'The only real valuable thing is intuition,' and that most of his innovation was just good guesswork. This association of reason with the fanciful seems an incredible contradiction – science and parapsychology (which intuition is) have traditionally been in separate camps. But research is now showing that our world is far more complex and multilay-ered than previously thought, and within those layers is room for intuition. Indeed research has also shown that intuition or instinct is far more informed and rational than originally thought, and can often be as good a judge as slow deliberation.

Before we look at what exactly is going on when we ex-perience intuition and how we can fine-tune our ability to make the best use of it, let's look at some examples of intuition:

We walk into a room full of people and are introduced to someone who is apparently liked and well respected. We take an immediate and instinctive dislike to that person for no obvious reason. Later – perhaps a lot later – our initial judgement is proved correct when some-thing is revealed about the person or their behaviour. Conversely, we may immediately warm to someone on first meeting and they become our lifelong friend.

You are asked to make a decision, but what you instinc-tively feel to be the right decision is not the most logical or rational one.

You instinctively take a different route home, catch a different bus or train, or postpone a trip, and later find out that by doing so you avoided an accident. Whenever a plane crashes there is someone who should have been on the plane but changed their flight at the last moment because of a premonition.

You make a minor, spur-of-the-moment change to your plans that has a significant knock-on effect on the rest of your life.

As well as Albert Einstein there are many other famous examples of people who have achieved a great deal by acting on their intuition. Here are a few:

Ray Kroc went against his financial advisor's advice and followed his instinct in 1960 when he borrowed $2.7 million and bought out the franchise of McDonald's and turned it into the most successful fast food operation in the world.

Sir Richard Branson, who started out in his teens selling records from the boot of his car and became a multi-millionaire from his business enterprises, says he makes a decision about a person or business venture within thirty seconds of meeting the person or reading the business proposal. His instincts have clearly served him very well: a recent estimate put his fortune at £1.5 billion ($2.5 billion)!

Conrad Hilton, founder of the Hilton hotel chain, claims he often relies on hunches. For example, he wanted a property in New York that was being sold through sealed (secret) bids. At the last minute, on a hunch, he changed his bid from $159,000 to $174,000 and thereby secured the property. The next highest bid had been $173,000. He later sold the property for several million dollars.

Felix Dennis, who started work as a gravedigger, made a fortune in Britain from publishing. In his book *How to Get Rich*, he says he ignores sound advice from his directors, lawyers and accountants and goes with his gut instincts. At the last count he was worth £500 million.

Following instincts isn't only about making money. Jonas Salk discovered the polio vaccine after spotting a flaw in a medical lecture at college. He later said, 'The light went on at that point. Intuition tells the thinking mind where to look next.'

And possibly the most famous incident of intuition was that of the racing car driver Juan Fangio. He was racing at the 1950 Monaco Grand Prix and instinctively braked as he approached a blind corner, unaware there'd been a serious accident round the corner, which he would have driven straight into. He couldn't possibly have seen round the corner but had gone with his instinct to brake sharply, which very likely saved his life.

These examples show that intuition is a very good asset. So what is actually happening to allow us what appears to be a magical or extrasensory power, and is it something we can develop? To answer this, first let us look at what researchers now believe happens when we experience intuition.

A good place to start is with the above example of the Argentinean racing driver Juan Fangio, who apparently had a sixth sense that he should brake. Here lies the key to understanding intuition. Picture the scene at the Grand Prix. Juan Fangio is racing around the circuit, foot hard on the accelerator, focused and intent on winning. The stadium is packed and the audience is watching the race with bated breath. Juan Fangio races along the straight and then towards the blind bend, beyond which there is a pile-up he cannot see. It is a disaster waiting to happen. But at the last second, instead of continuing round the bend and ploughing headlong into the other cars, to the amazement of those watching, Fangio brakes fiercely, thereby avoiding the accident and saving himself. Afterwards Fangio said he didn't know why he'd braked: the decision to brake had been instinctive, and went against all his other thoughts of winning the race.

Fangio's apparently amazing foresight was captured on camera and psychologists were very keen to investigate what appeared to be a first-class example of the sixth sense or intuition at work. Fangio agreed to do some work with the psychologists and together they analysed the CCTV tapes of the race. To begin with it looked as though Fangio had indeed had some dramatic intuitive perception, so startling was the evidence. But on further examination the tapes revealed something very interesting. The tapes showed Fangio's car racing towards the blind bend but they also showed the audience in the stadium. The audience had a good view of the other side of the bend where the accident was, and they were looking not at Fangio's car but at the pile-up. Fangio couldn't possibly have consciously seen the audience: he was going so fast they would have been a blur. But subconsciously he had seen them and the looks on their faces as they saw the pile-up. In that split second, his brain, using his previous experience of racing, had interpreted their expressions as a sign of danger. It was this that had caused Fangio to brake.

It therefore appears intuition is not a sixth sense but that in a split second our brain subconsciously assesses external cues – i.e. what is going on around us – and processes these in the light of our previous experience. It then makes a decision and sends a message to our conscious brain which we perceive as intuition. Or to put it another way the brain is doing what it normally does – taking in and processing information and using it to make a decision – but with intuition it happens so fast we're not aware of it.

Another more frequent, yet no less incredible, example of intuition is that of experienced firefighters. When firefighters are working in a blazing building they often experience an intuitive feeling or gut reaction that tells them when to get out of the building – a few seconds before a floor gives way or a wall crashes, for example – so saving themselves and their team. This intuition is based on years of experience from fighting fires in similar situations. So while the firefighters are concentrating on fighting the fire their brains are subconsciously picking up and processing all the external cues: changes in flame height or direction, a shift in the wind, a new draft, a stillness in the air, a sudden unidentified noise, etc. Their brains' subconscious compares all these cues to their previous experiences of firefighting and make a decision on when it is time to get out. Obviously firefighters also make many conscious decisions on how to fight fires, but time and time again firefighters recount how they relied on gut instinct to abandon a blazing building and get out.

Likewise the 'gut reaction' we feel when we meet someone for the first time and either take an immediate dislike to them or instinctively warm to them is based on our brain receiving cues and assessing them in the light of our previous experience of people. As we are politely shaking hands and smiling at the person our subconscious is busy comparing their handshake, smile, eye contact, body language, etc. with our massive database of meeting other people, and then draws a conclusion. This is all done in a split second.

The decision to drive home by a different route for no obvious reason which resulted in our missing a bad accident was probably not the result of the incredible sixth sense or good luck as we thought it was. While leaving the office that night and walking to the car our senses were picking up many external cues which our subconscious processed – the weather, a snippet of a radio announcement from a passing car, a glimpse of a newspaper headline, the unusually heavy traffic – all of which were compared to our previous driving experience. Our brain subconsciously recognized that driving conditions on our usual route were likely to be hazardous and best avoided, so we chose a different route.

Although research is ongoing into how often intuition makes a better judgement than a reasoned conscious decision, and while some people seem to be naturally more intuitive than others, we can all benefit from listening to our inner voice of instinct. For as we have seen intuition is not a random feeling or hocus-pocus but an incredible subconscious burst of logical thinking.

How to make the best of your intuition

Here are a few tips:

1. Trust in your intuition. It is your subconscious mind helping out your conscious mind by processing information at phenomenal speed. Trust it and go with it. Experienced chess players don't play just by analysing the pieces and logically working out moves. They hold thousands of patterns of chess moves in their subconscious and rely on the subconscious providing the right move. Have faith in your intuition so that if, for example, you are interviewing candidates for a job, look at their qualifications, listen to what they have to say at the interview, and harness your 'gut feeling' as to who is the best person for the job.

I sit on adoption panels whose purpose is to assess and approve those who want to adopt. Prospective adopters will have spent over two years being thoroughly vetted and assessed by a social worker; coming before the panel is the final hurdle before being approved and then adopting a child who needs a home. Recently, one couple who came before a panel I was sitting on seemed ideal candidates. They were in their early thirties, had a stable relationship, were aware of the issues facing adopted children and gave all the right answers to the questions the panel put to them. As is usual practice, they were asked to leave the room while the panel discussed their application. The panel consisted of ten, and eight of my colleagues were in favour of approving the couple, but I and one other person had reservations. For reasons we couldn't properly explain my colleague and I felt the couple weren't as committed as they appeared. We deliberated for half an hour (not unusual for an adoption panel) and my colleague and I were finally persuaded to go with the majority view – that the couple should be allowed to adopt.

Just as the chairperson was about to call the couple back into the room and tell them the good news, a knock sounded on the door. The couple's social worker appeared, looking very embarrassed. She said she was very sorry but the couple had decided to withdraw their application as they had decided to try for a child of their own through IVF (in vitro fertilization). She was as shocked as anyone, as she had spent two years working with and assessing the couple and had had no doubt as to their commitment. Clearly my colleague and I, using our previous experience, had picked up non-verbal cues about the couple's lack of commitment, though we couldn't have said what these were.

2. Go with your first response. If you are faced with a decision, whether it is which dish to choose from a menu at a restaurant, which dress, sofa or car to buy, or which of two equally appealing job offers you should accept, then go with your first response. This choice will have been made as a result of previous experience and information which your brain has processed and stored. Intuition won't always provide a solution when you are faced with a decision and often you will have to plough through conscious reasoning before you can make the decision, but when intuition obligingly provides you with the answer, take it and be grateful: your subconscious has saved you a lot of work.

3. Be creative. It is thought that intuition comes from the right side of the brain, which is where creativity flourishes. As I have already mentioned, creative people tend to be more intuitive, but the rest of us can catch up. To help strengthen your intuition, try new creative pastimes – writing, painting, dancing (alone if you don't feel like joining a class or going clubbing), acting, landscaping your garden, redesigning a room, listening to music or better still playing a musical instrument. Anything that lifts you out of conscious thought to *feel* rather than think is creative and will develop your intuition.

4. Sleep on it. Sleep can encourage intuition. However, interpreting dreams should be treated with caution. There are many books claiming to interpret dreams but generally dreams are nature's way of dealing with life experience – the subconscious cleansing the psyche ready for the next day. The answer to a problem may come in a dream but is more likely to come the following day after a good night's sleep. The expression 'I'll sleep on it' has real meaning, for often a solution that had perversely escaped us one day miraculously appears the next morning. It seems that while we sleep our subconscious mind processes information, forms ideas and makes decisions. Also the semi-awake state – as you drift into sleep or slowly surface from it – is a time when ideas are freed from the subconscious. If it is not practical for you to take the time to 'sleep on it', then try simply relaxing (with your eyes closed if possible) and letting your mind float free. Not only will this recharge your energy levels but it will open the pathway from your conscious mind to your subconscious. If an idea or solution pops into your mind while you are in this relaxed state, give it serious consideration, for it is likely to be a flash of insight.

Einstein summed up the relationship between conscious reasoning and intuition beautifully: *The intuitive mind is a*

sacred gift and the rational mind is a faithful servant. We have
created a society that honours the servant and has forgotten the
gift. So make the most of your mind on all levels, for it is
truly a complex and wondrous gift.

CHAPTER TWELVE

Create a Positive Environment

A positive environment is crucial if we are to be happy and contented and get the very best from life. Environment in this context means our home and workplace, and the people in our lives. You may think you have little choice or control in these matters – for example, the tiny flat you rent and can't afford to move from. If so, you'll be surprised at just how much choice you do have. If necessary, you can make many changes so that your environment is positive and complements the person you are.

Home environment

We'll start with the easy bit – your home environment, which is crucial to your well-being.

Home can be anything from a shared bedsit to a mansion. Whatever you think of as home is your home environment, regardless of its size or location. It is the place where you live: go to at the end of the day to escape from the outside world; relax in the evenings and weekends; invite family and friends to; and usually sleep in. It is your own personal space, your nest, and for you to be contented there it needs to be user friendly and at one with the person you are. It should generate warmth and happiness and be a place you can relax in and be yourself.

Whatever your home environment, make it yours; give it your stamp of approval so that it complements and expresses your personality and you feel at one with it. You can achieve this through the furnishings and the objects with which you surround yourself – for example, pictures, candles, ornaments, potted plants and general objets d'art – and through the colour scheme you choose. Just as the colour of our clothes reflects or even alters our mood, so the colours in our homes should be in tune with us – how we see ourselves and want others to see us.

* Red, orange and yellow suggest warmth, comfort, excitement and energy.
* Pale green (very popular at present) is relaxing and symbolizes nature.
* Pale blue is calming.
* Dark blue suggests strength and steadfastness.
* Lavender suggests refinement, grace and elegance.

* Light grey is a neutral colour, often favoured by men, and suggests someone cool and conservative, seldom evoking strong emotion (but dark grey can be seen as moody).

Check that the colours of your home reflect the person you are and if you are unhappy with them then change them – by redecorating, for instance. A pot of paint is relatively cheap and you will feel its benefit for years.

If you share a house or room you will obviously have to discuss the colour scheme, furnishings, etc. with those you live with and decide on something that suits you all. But even if you have to compromise on your choice in the communal areas to keep everyone happy, somewhere within the house, flat or room will be a small area that is truly yours to do with as you wish. This may be your half of the bedroom you share, your bed, the area where you relax and listen to music, read or watch television or even a favourite armchair nestled in a corner. Whatever you see as your place, decorate it to suit you with colours and objects that complement your personality. Cushions, a throw-over rug, a lamp, framed photographs, a personalized mug or towel, etc. can work wonders. Touches such as these will create your space, an environment where you can relax, be yourself and recharge your batteries at the end of the day.

Teenagers are especially good at marking out and personalizing their space, which is often their bedroom or part of a bedroom. If teenagers share a bedroom it is obvious as soon as you walk into the room where one person's space ends and the next begins without any physical boundary lines.

> When teenagers come into care they often arrive with all their personal possessions in one suitcase, but within hours he or she will have claimed their bedroom (or part of the bedroom if they share) with posters and pictures on the walls, photographs, books, DVDs, Nintendo games on the shelves and soft toys and clothes arranged or strewn around the room. It can look quite a mess to the untrained eye, but care workers know how important it is for the young person to mark out and personalize their territory so that they have a place to call home.

Home is not about the space we occupy but the 'feel' of the space. Henry Van Dyke (1852–1933), an American author, educator and clergyman, put it nicely:

> Every house where love abides
> And friendship is a guest,
> Is surely home, and home sweet home
> For there the heart can rest.

Which leads nicely to:

How to live with others

• •

Although the number of single-person households is rising across the developed world (at present 30 per cent in UK and Western Europe, 22 per cent in Eastern Europe, 26.7 per cent in the USA, 25.7 per cent in Australasia) the majority of adults share their home with others. This may be a partner, husband or wife, parents, extended family or friends. It is often said that you don't truly know someone until you live with them, meaning you will only discover their bad habits when you live together. Much patience, sensitivity, empathy, understanding and negotiation on everyone's part are needed for adults to successfully live together. Living in a household with children is somewhat different, as the children will be expected to conform to certain norms and boundaries for their behaviour, put in place by the adults who are raising them (see my book *Happy Kids*, HarperCollins, 2010). But if you are an adult living with other adults, here are a few simple rules to help make your home environment happy for everyone:

1. Agree on each individual's personal space – for example, their bedroom – and respect their privacy. Do not enter their space unless you are invited.

2. Don't listen to other's telephone conversations, read their mail, texts and emails or generally pry. The person will tell you what he or she wants you to know and the rest is private.

3. Communicate. Listen and talk to those you live with.

4. Don't gossip about other household members. Distrust brings down a household quicker than anything.

5. Air grievances calmly and before they build up.

6. Agree on cost sharing: who is responsible for paying for what. Have a kitty for communal commodities – for example, toilet paper, soap and washing-up liquid. Agree an amount to pay in and make sure everyone pays.

7. Agree on a rota for household chores and stick to the agreement. Most arguments in respect of this arise as a result of one person feeling 'put upon', i.e. doing the majority of the housework.

8. Respect communal areas: for example, don't hog the bathroom at 8.oo a.m. when everyone is trying to get ready and leave for work, or leave nail clippings in the sink, or pubic hair in the shower. In showing respect for the communal areas you are showing respect for the other members of your household.

9. Be considerate about the noise you make whether it is your music, television, mobile phone or coming home late at night. Your noise may be pleasant to you but others may feel very differently.

10. Show little acts of kindness, for example by offering to make a household member a cup of tea when they arrive home from work exhausted and you are in first. Kindness costs nothing but the rewards are priceless.

11. Forgive others. No one is perfect.

By following these simple rules your home environment will be peaceful and an asset to you.

Work environment

Equally important as a happy home environment is a good work environment. You will probably be spending much of your week at work, so your workplace needs to feel comfortable, reflecting who you are, as well as being conducive to your work productivity. Those of us who are homemakers or work from home will find it easier to create a positive working environment, as there won't be the same constraints from office regulations or the preferences of colleagues.

If you are a homemaker, possibly raising children or caring for elderly parents, with no work outside the home, then view the whole house as your work environment (as well as your home). If you work from home – i.e. your work is sourced from outside the home, but you largely do it at home – then you should either have a study or a dedicated space for work. Treat this space as your work environment so that when you enter it you feel positive about 'going to work'. It might only be a corner of a room, but decorate your study or workspace so that you are happy to be at work. Choose your chair, desk (or table), lighting, etc. to suit you so you feel comfortable and can concentrate.

Those of us who go to a place of work can still create a convivial working environment that is user friendly and personalized, despite the constraints. A potted plant, a small vase of fresh flowers, a family photograph or an ornament on your desk or nearby shelf or windowsill are very effective. Likewise your choice of mouse mat, pen, coffee mug, etc. all help create a working environment that is tailormade to your individual self. If you're an office worker, make sure your chair is comfortable. This is important both for your physical and mental well-being: research has shown that employees who are comfortable and happy at work are far more productive, unsurprisingly. Position filing cabinets and other office furniture to enhance your workspace, not make you feel caged in.

Even if you share your workspace with many others – if you work, for example, in an open-plan office, supermarket or school – there are many small things you can do to make your work environment pleasant and personal. Teachers usually have their own pen sets and a few personal items

– for example, a fancy paperweight on their desk at the front of the classroom, and their own coffee mug in the staff room; long-distance lorry drivers adorn their cabs with all manner of memorabilia from places they have visited; the furnishings and decoration of rest rooms in large stores or offices are usually designed by a committee of employees. Even toilet attendants, working in one of the least inviting of environments, can create a positive working environment by keeping it sparkling clean, smelling sweetly and with a vase of fresh flowers.

Just as you are likely to spend more of your waking hours in your work environment than in your home, so you are likely to spend more time with your work colleagues than with your family and friends. Even if you enjoy a positive working relationship with all your colleagues, and your personalities are compatible, there will still be times when you disagree. It is vital you smooth over any disagreements quickly; otherwise going to work will be a negative experience for you, and your work will suffer. It has been said that working with a colleague you don't get along with is like a bad marriage but without the option of divorce. There is also the issue of the workplace bully who, recent research suggests, is far more prevalent than previously thought: 80 per cent of workers in the UK are aware of bullying in their workplace.

Whatever your status or work situation, here are the golden rules for creating a positive and harmonious working environment so that you are happy and contented at work:

1. Take pride in your work and do it to the best of your ability. That is what you are paid for.

2. If you have a grievance, pursue it through the appropriate channel. Don't moan to colleagues.

3. Don't gossip about others. News travels fast at work and if you gossip no one will trust you.

4. Avoid discussing emotive topics with your colleagues, for example politics and religion.

5. When you start a new job, spend time getting to know the workplace and your colleagues rather than rushing in like 'a new broom'. Even senior management should spend time getting the feel of their new position before making changes.

6. Don't change what works.

7. Be polite to everyone, from the cleaner to the managing director. Good manners cost you nothing, but bad manners will cost you respect from others and even your job. Say please and thank you and hold doors open for colleagues.

8. Respect and praise your colleagues for their skills, knowledge and achievements, but don't patronize or grovel.

9. Deal with others' mistakes sensitively and quietly. Make any criticism constructive.

10. Admit to your own mistakes.

11. If you are criticized or disciplined for good reason, accept it as positive feedback. We all make mistakes and errors of judgement. Apologize for your error and reassure that it won't happen again.

12. Dress appropriately for your role and work situation. If in doubt, err on the side of sobriety.

13. Deal with the workplace bully as follows. First try ignoring them: they may get fed up and leave you alone. If they don't, try putting them in their place with a few sharp remarks. If the bullying persists, report the bully to the appropriate person. Bullying is unacceptable at work, just as it is at school.

14. If you are ill, don't go into work; you are unlikely to be very productive and no one will thank you for spreading germs.

15. Respect other's privacy and space. Don't read their mail or emails or look over their shoulder at their computer screen unless they ask you to. And obviously don't rummage through their desk, drawers, locker, etc.

16. Clean up after yourself in communal areas, for example the rest room.

17. Don't cause offence by talking loudly, chewing gum, burping, farting or doing anything else that is likely to bother others. Work situations often require that we are physically close to a colleague, so remember good personal hygiene.

18. Be grateful you have a job; many don't. If you really don't like your work, then take steps to find another job. Life is too short to be unhappy.

CHAPTER THIRTEEN

Reduce Stress

In my role as a foster carer I meet stress almost on a daily basis: children and young people stressed and confused by being brought into care; their parents, stressed and angry at having their children taken away; my family, stressed and upset by hearing and dealing with the situations these children, their families, social workers and the system place upon us. As is the case with most foster carers, my family and I have had to develop strategies to deal with the stress; otherwise we wouldn't function.

In my role as a writer I've received thousands of emails from adults and young people around the world who confide that they are stressed and ask for my advice and help. The causes of being stressed are many and include bereavement, forthcoming exams, past and present abuse, a challenging child, a failing relationship and conditions such as anorexia, agoraphobia, OCD (obsessive compulsive disorder) and self harming. While a little stress, which gets the adrenaline flowing and motivates us, is good, being stressed for long periods, for any reason, is at best counter-productive and at worst life threatening. Scientific research has found a causal link between on-going high levels of stress and an increased risk of having a stroke or heart attack.

Most of us living in the developed world will experience stress on a daily basis and for many of us the level of stress will be unhealthily high, making us, tired, irritable and depressed, and ultimately causing physical and mental health problems. Being able to deal with stress successfully is therefore crucial for our physical and mental well-being, happiness and contentment.

It is obviously appropriate that we feel stressed at times of crisis – bereavement, divorce, moving house or changing job, etc. – but often our stress levels are out of proportion to the actual situation. The level of stress we feel is based on a number of factors, including our personality, our work and home situation, our existing stress levels and the support we perceive we receive from others. An already over-stretched single mother, for example, may go to pieces if she drops an egg while cooking breakfast and trying to get her young children to school on time. Someone with more time and support, on the other hand, and with a calmer disposition, would deal with the accident more philosophically, possibly even laughing at their clumsiness.

Children can feel stress as much as adults but show it in different ways, for example through challenging behaviour, bed-wetting, sleeping or eating disorders, or becoming quiet and withdrawn. I talk about childhood stress in my book *Happy Kids*.

But it isn't all doom and gloom, for although we can't completely remove stressful situations from our lives (they are often out of our control), we can change the way we react to them, greatly reducing the level of stress we experience and making us feel less stressed. Before we look at techniques for doing this it might be helpful to look at what happens in our bodies when we are stressed.

Believe it or not, the symptoms of stress are nature's way of protecting us from danger by preparing our bodies to deal with it. A long time ago when we lived in caves danger was all around us, especially in the form of attack by wild animals. Then our only options were to stay and fight for our lives or run for safety: fight or flight. Although it is now unlikely we will be in danger of attack from wild animals, we still experience threats, or stress. While these threats are of a different type, if we feel threatened our minds and bodies react now in the same way as our ancestors' did. To prepare our bodies for fight or flight, hormones including adrenaline and cortisol are released into the bloodstream, with the following immediate effects:

* our heart rate, breathing and blood supply increase (so that we can run faster or fight harder)
* our pupils dilate (allowing us to see more)
* our alertness increases and reaction time improves (so we react more quickly)
* we sweat more (to keep us cool)
* our pain threshold and muscle tone increase (increasing our endurance)

* our digestive system shuts down (the energy usually used for digestion is redirected to our muscles).

We are all familiar with the racing heart, sweaty hands, dry mouth and heightened state of alert we experience when we are stressed.

The problem comes because modern-day stress is not caused by threats that require us to run or fight for our lives, and therefore we do not need adrenaline and the other hormones – originally lifesavers – in order to deal with them. Modern-day threats are largely 'passive' and include:

* money worries
* marriage or relationship problems
* unrealistic expectations – at home and work
* unemployment
* too many tasks and not enough time
* too much responsibility
* lack of control – at home or work
* lack of support.

All these situations are likely to be chronic and ongoing and not resolved by running away or physically fighting. Nevertheless the unneeded stress hormones remain present in the body, causing high blood pressure, weakened immune system and ultimately physical and mental illness. While we can't stop our bodies reacting to stress any more than we can remove all situations that cause us stress, we can reduce the amount of stress in our lives, and so help ourselves towards happiness and contentment.

How not to feel stressed

Despite the challenges of fostering (and bringing up my family alone), my life is not stressful, but it used to be; indeed my stress levels at one time were getting out of hand. They peaked about fifteen years ago (when my husband left me), resulting in sleepless nights, unexplained skin rashes, irritability, permanent anxiety and an overriding feeling that I couldn't cope. I was fostering a challenging teenager at the time and my own children, who were very young, were obviously upset by their father leaving and understandably needed a lot of reassurance. I felt the pressure build all around me.

Once the teenager had returned home to live I took a break from fostering to concentrate on my family and me. I slowed the pace and began addressing all the issues that result from divorce, practical (trying to pay the bills etc.) and emotional (feelings of rejection). By the end of six months although I was still hurting from my husband leaving I was far less stressed. I had got my life (and my family's) back on track and felt ready to foster again.

Although I didn't know it at the time, the techniques I used for dealing with stress were already acknowledged to be good strategies for stress reduction that had been shown to work. These are the same strategies I pass on to readers who email saying they are stressed and asking for help. Some of them will sound familiar (from reading this book so far), for the strategies we use for reducing stress overlap with and complement the techniques we use for leading a positive, happy and contented life.

1. Identify the source of your stress. The reasons for your feeling stressed won't always be obvious, but it is very important you find the source; this is a crucial first step. If you are divorcing or moving house, or have lost your job, for example, the source will be clear, but often we cannot see a cause, so we generalize:

'I'm so stressed.'

'My life is one long stress.'

'I'm stressed out all the time.'

This won't be true: no one is permanently stressed. There will be a source – a root cause. The problem with generalizing is that it encourages the stress to grow. Sometimes the root cause turns out to be relatively small but the stress has spread to other aspects of our life because it hasn't been identified and dealt with. Here are some examples of stress that often go unidentified and therefore fester:

* a badly behaving child or teenager
* an unreasonable workload
* unreasonable pressure from others
* money problems
* disputes with family, friends or work colleagues
* sexual difficulties
* a new baby
* marriage, a new relationship, stepchildren
* chronic guilt, anger or frustration
* striving for perfection in ourselves or others
* fear of failing or being deserted.

There are many more and it may be that you find more than one cause, but once you have identified the source(s) of your stress you will be well on the way to reducing or even eliminating the feelings it is causing.

2. Examine the cause of the stress. Examine the source of stress closely and break it down into its various parts. By doing this you will be able to see exactly what needs to change.

Let's say the cause of your stress is the care of an elderly relative, a huge ongoing commitment that has become very stressful. Examine your role. What exactly is it about caring for your relative that is stressing you? The time it takes to wash, dress or feed her? The laundry her incontinence generates? The call on your time? Her constant demands or moaning? Her ingratitude? The cause of your stress won't be everything about caring for her, I can assure you; indeed, once you examine your role you will find there is much about caring for her that you enjoy and makes you feel good.

When you have pinpointed the trigger for your stress you can deal with it. For example, if the trigger is the call on your time, then examine what it is that is taking the most time and work out ways to reduce it. It may be the amount of laundry you are doing for the lady. If so, is it possible to send it to a launderette? Are you eligible for a grant to cover this? And so on.

I receive many emails from readers saying how stressed they are by their child or children's behaviour – so many in fact that I was persuaded to write a book to help, *Happy Kids*. I always start by asking these parents which aspect of their child or children's behaviour is causing them stress. They often reply, 'All of it!' So I say, 'Even when they sleep?' This starts them thinking, and the process of identifying which part of their child's behaviour is causing the problem. Once they have identified this I suggest strategies for changing the child's behaviour so that parent and child can enjoy a stress-free relationship. As with all stress, once you have found the root cause of the problem it can be dealt with, and the stress reduced or even eliminated.

3. Learn to say no. This is essential when reducing stress. Decide on what you can reasonably do, and say no to what you can't. A polite refusal is far better than feeling stressed by an unreasonable burden of responsibility. Learn to say no at work and home; do what you can but don't take on tasks and responsibilities that place an unrealistic burden on your time. If you work as a builder, for example, as well as having a young family, it is highly unlikely you will have time to build your neighbour's extension in your spare time, no matter how nicely he or she asks you. Rather than taking on the whole project in addition to your other responsibilities, it is more realistic for you to give your neighbour some advice and encouragement. Likewise, if you are a full-time mum with a young family it is quite possible you may have to say no to your best friend or sister when she asks you to look after her two children every Friday so that she can play badminton or go to bingo. So often we agree to do something because we are kind, want to help and don't like to say no. But saying a polite *No, I'm sorry, I can't* will gain you more respect than agreeing and then struggling under the additional responsibility. It will also save you a lot of stress.

4. Take time for yourself. This is essential. Regardless of how busy you are, find a few hours each week and make them yours – 'me time'. If you can't find those hours in your week then examine your commitments and let something go. No one is so indispensable (not even the Prime Minister or President) that they can't take a few hours out of their schedule to indulge themselves. This will be your time to do with as you choose – pursue a hobby, go for a walk, swim, learn to play a musical instrument, meet a friend for a drink or coffee, read a book, visit a spa, have a massage or simply watch a DVD. Taking time for yourself not only de-stresses you but allows you space to get in touch again with yourself – the person you are – which can very easily become lost beneath a hectic lifestyle. In the same vein, take a holiday – if possible by going away. Nothing de-stresses faster than removing oneself from the routine and responsibilities of everyday life, even for a weekend.

5. Examine your average day. Are you running to stand still? as the saying goes. If so, scale down your 'to do' list. As mentioned above, if you find it difficult to make a few hours yours each week, then you are doing too much. Let something go.

> Bob and Sandra were a couple I used to know who were the ultimate Supermum and Superdad. They both worked full time while raising their three children; were accomplished DIY enthusiasts (their house was immaculate); had their elderly relatives for the day on alternate Sundays; volunteered for everything that was asked of them – PTA, Neighbourhood Watch, charity collections, town carnival, etc. – and still had time to throw parties. They put many of us to shame with the amount they achieved. But behind the scenes it was a different matter. With no time to relax or for each other they were constantly bickering, and they were frequently ill, with an ongoing list of minor ailments including coughs, colds and stomach upsets, etc.

Things came to a head one Christmas when Bob agreed to help out on Christmas Day in a soup kitchen for the homeless. While this was very noble of him, it left Sandra entertaining their eighteen guests alone for the whole day. Come dinnertime when the turkey wasn't quite done but the vegetables were, Sandra snapped, and to the amazement of all her guests she broke down in floods of tears and confessed her life was so stressful she couldn't go on any more.

Her brother sensibly put a large drink in her hand and sent her into the sitting room to rest while everyone else helped prepare the meal. Dinner was served (albeit a little late) with all the guests in very good spirits having had a great time helping, while Sandra admitted it was her best Christmas ever. I would like to say that this was the turning point for Sandra and Bob and that they slowed their pace and led less stressful lives, but once Christmas was over they continued as before and came to view Sandra's breakdown on Christmas Day as a minor blip because she hadn't been 'feeling too well'. Sadly by not learning to say no they continued to lead stressful lives.

6. Be positive. In earlier chapters we saw that thinking and acting positively are a crucial part of leading a happy and contented life. Thinking and acting positively are also fundamental to living a stress-free life, as stress is *always* a result of negative thoughts. If you don't believe me, then try and think of a situation where you were stressed and had positive thoughts. You can't. Even if your stress was a result of a proposed enjoyable experience – for example, arranging a children's birthday party or going on holiday – your stress will have been caused by worrying about possible negative outcomes, i.e. fixating on what could go wrong with the party or holiday. Such worries are often 'What if?' questions – *What if I miss the plane/forget to pack something? What if no one comes to my child's party? What if I'm ill?*

I guarantee you will not be able to find a situation stressful if you think and act positively. So next time you find your stress levels rising, whether at the thought of a situation in the future or because of something that is already taking place, change your negative thoughts to positive ones, and then continue with a positive act.

In the case of your child's birthday party, to which you fear no one will come, you can say, *Of course lots of children will come to my daughter's party; she has many friends. I need to make lots of jellies and cakes*, and then start baking.

Or it might be that you are at work and about to deliver a presentation to the board, feeling your stress levels rise because the board opposed your plans the last time. Tell yourself that a little stress is fine because you are excited by what you are about to say, and of course the board will accept your suggestion because it's the best idea proposed in ages. If your thoughts jump back to the negative and the last time you were before the board, switch them back to the positive and the great idea you are now suggesting. Then take a deep breath and, concentrating solely on the merits of your proposal, look at the members of the board and start talking.

And don't forget your sense of humour and to smile. Appropriate humour de-stresses not only you but also those around you. When you smile, all those tiny facial muscles send signals to your brain to tell you you are happy. It is impossible to be stressed and happy at the same time, so smile away.

7. Be philosophical. Earlier we looked at developing an attitude that focuses on the positive and makes light of the negative. Well, that same philosophy keeps stress from our lives. Just as being philosophical about life's little downers helps keep us happy and contented, so being philosophical allows us to view potentially stressful situations differently and defuses them, stopping them from being stressful. If a situation has the potential to cause stress, or has already gone less well than you'd hoped and become stressful, then view it philosophically:

It could have been worse.

Every cloud has a silver lining.

Oh well, tomorrow is another day.

It's all part of life's rich tapestry etc.

Saying to yourself *I will do my best, accept what I can't change and not try to control what isn't mine* is another good philosophy.

8. Express your feelings. Keeping your feelings to yourself has the potential to allow them to build up and stress you, until eventually, like Sandra, you can't take any more and you break down. Don't bottle up your feelings. Express how you feel appropriately – in a rational and calm manner and to an appropriate person. I say more about this in Chapter Fifteen.

9. Let go of anger. At the very beginning of this book – the first step to being truly happy and contented – I explained the need to let go of anger. Stress and anger go hand in hand. You may be angry for any number of reasons: for example, because someone has treated you badly; as a result of a situation, for example bereavement; or maybe you are angry with yourself for doing something really silly or acting out of character. Whatever the cause of your anger, it will make you feel stressed, and in order to remove the stress it is causing you will need to let go of it (see Chapter One). Not only will you feel relieved, happier and contented but also your levels of stress chemicals will automatically fall. If you can forgive – others or yourself – then do so; otherwise just let go and move on.

A quick de-stress

So far we have looked at techniques for reducing our overall and long-term stress levels. Now let us look at techniques for calming yourself if you find yourself in a stressful situation. You know the symptoms – racing heart, sweaty palms, feeling hot and cold at the same time. Panic has set in, fear has taken over and you are at the mercy of your body. Maybe you are running very late; going to a job interview; speaking at an important meeting; do not have enough time to meet a crucial deadline; meeting your ex-partner to discuss contact arrangements for your children; or dealing with an angry and aggressive customer. In such situations what we need is a quick-fix solution. The following will achieve this – three simple steps, all done at the same time to calm and de-stress:

1. Take a deep breath slowly in and then out. This is an old and well-practised technique for calming the body and mind, and there is a good reason why it works. As we've seen, when we are stressed hormones make our mind and body ready for fight or flight. The result is that the heart and lungs work faster as they pump more oxygen around the body, ready for action, and our muscles tighten, making our breathing shallow – just the opposite of what the body needs. Taking a deep breath gives the body the oxygen it needs, counteracting this effect.

2. Relax your muscles. At the same time as taking a deep breath, unclench your hands and jaw, uncurl your toes, lower your shoulders and relax your spine. This will relax your contracted muscles and you will instantly feel calmer and less stressed.

3. Refocus. When we are stressed we tend to focus on objects close by, as our world contracts to us and our fear. We need to gain a better perspective. As you take the deep breath and relax your muscles, raise your head and look as far as possible into the distance. If you are in a room with a window, glance out of the window and look as far as you can see. If there is no window, look at the furthest point in the room. If you are outside, look as far as you can into the distance – to the horizon or sky. Redirecting the vision opens our world and puts our situation into a better perspective, minimizing our panic and stress.

The above technique is simple: take a deep breath, relax your muscles and refocus. It takes no more than five seconds and, unlike many relaxation techniques, is instant. No one will know what you are doing; you can use it anywhere – when you are driving, at an interview, in a meeting, dealing with aggressive people, etc. I use it whenever I face a situation I know from past experience might cause me anxiety or stress: examples from fostering include giving evidence in court, meeting hostile parents of a child I am fostering, accompanying a young person to a police interview, very large formal meetings, etc. I have a quick de-stress as I enter the situation and at any time during the situation when I feel my anxiety levels rise.

I recommended this technique to a young teacher who was in her first post, teaching maths to fourteen-year-olds in an inner-city school. Halfway through the term she was so stressed by the bad behaviour of the unruly classes, that she was thinking of handing in her notice and quitting teaching altogether. She said she could feel her stress levels rise before she'd even entered the classroom, and she was sure some of the pupils picked up on her fear and played her up even more. This was quite possible, as fear is tangible. I suggested she use the technique before going into the classroom and also at any time she felt herself becoming stressed during lessons. I also included some strategies for controlling the class (see *Happy Kids*).

She emailed me after a couple of weeks and said that although teaching some of the classes was still an uphill struggle and she wondered how much some of the pupils were actually learning, she felt more in control of the classes' behaviour and was certainly less stressed.

By practising the techniques for stress reduction in this chapter we can reduce or even eliminate both long-term and short-term stress. We therefore owe it to ourselves to aim for a stress-free life, which will assist our journey to lasting happiness and contentment.

CHAPTER FOURTEEN

Live in the Present

I receive many emails that include words such as these:

I only wish I'd appreciated what I had at the time.

I wished I'd realized that then.

If I had my time over again …

Where did my life go?

These are from readers who, in some way, regret the past and not making the most of life at the time. I fully appreciate their lament, for it is so easy to spend too much time planning for and worrying about the future, and not enough time appreciating the present.

It seems to be part of the developed world's philosophy to plan ahead. We are constantly bombarded by advertising to persuade us to invest in the future: insurance which matures in thirty years; long-term bonds with a high-interest return; pension plans; a discount if we book our annual holiday a year in advance; committing to a Christmas savings plan in January and so on. Of course we need to plan ahead to some degree. As well as saving a little for the future to ensure we are comfortable, we need to plan life choices sensibly – what and where to study, our career, when to start a family, etc.

Unfortunately, however, modern-day society seems so fixated with planning for the future that the present falls into second place and can pass unnoticed. I feel very sad (and gloomy) when I receive emails from young people in their teens and early twenties who have their futures mapped out right down to the age at which they will retire. These young people will suddenly wake up in their forties and fifties and wonder where life went. I also fear they are setting themselves up for failure and will be very disappointed, for so often life doesn't deliver as planned. We need to be highly adaptable to accommodate life's changes; indeed, our long-term happiness and contentment rest on our willingness to adapt and change our plans (sometimes dramatically) when things don't work out as we'd hoped.

In order to get the very best from life we need to stop fixating and worrying about the future or fretting over the past. Torturing ourselves with a past mistake: *'If only I'd …'* – is negative and not compatible with a happy and contented lifestyle. Learn from past mistakes and then move on, and make the most of every minute by living in the here and now. Life isn't a rehearsal. We get only one go at it, so we need to make every moment count. This doesn't mean we should behave recklessly, or rush around every waking minute accomplishing, but whatever we are doing – whether it is compiling a report, reading, housework, taking the kids to school, DIY or simply relaxing in front of the television, we should enjoy it while we are doing it. This is the only way to fully appreciate and make the most of the precious gift of life.

How to live in the present

There are five simple rules for living in the present which, once mastered, will enable you to make the most of life and live every moment to the full.

1. Be aware. Take notice of your surroundings and your place in them. Connect with where you are and what you are doing. Use all your senses: see, hear, taste, smell and feel. Being aware of your surroundings – the smell of the early morning dew; the sight of the sun slowly turning the sky crimson as it creeps over the horizon; the sound of the unseen song thrush trilling in the tree; the taste of your toast in the morning; the familiar smell of your pillow as your head touches it at night – sets you firmly in the here and now. It becomes easier the more you do it, until it becomes second nature to feel and appreciate the wonder of the here and now.

> Many of the children I foster are so closed in upon themselves – either because they have been raised on television, PlayStation, etc., or because of abuse or neglect – that when I start helping them to connect by pointing out the simple pleasures that are all around them they are so excited that they go over the top. They tell me everything they see, hear, feel, touch and taste, all the time! It's as though a veil has suddenly been lifted and they are truly alive for the first time.

If you are someone who is not usually aware of their surroundings, then use all your senses to come alive and glory in the present.

2. Concentrate. Whatever you are doing, give it your full attention. If you are fully concentrating, you will accomplish unwelcome tasks more quickly, and pleasurable activities such as hobbies, socializing, going to the cinema or making love will be more pleasurable. You know the maxim: if something is worth doing it is worth doing well. To achieve your best you need to give it your full attention. If you are giving the task in hand your complete attention it is impossible not be in the present. Concentrating on whatever you are doing plants you firmly in the here and now.

As I sit writing at 6.00 a.m. (my writing time before my family wakes) I am aware – of the pen in my hand gliding over the paper, the silence around me, the smell and taste of my coffee – and I am completely focused on the words as I concentrate wholly on my writing.

3. Don't dwell on the future or the past. Acknowledge the past so that you can learn from your mistakes but then return to the present. Recognize your plans for the future and do what is necessary to set them in motion, but then come back to the here and now. Of course you can look forward to a holiday or some other pleasurable event, but try not to do so to the exclusion of the present. As soon as you catch yourself dwelling on the past or future, switch back to the present by becoming aware of what is around you. What can you see, hear, smell, touch or taste? This is the present, where life should be lived. The future is largely unpredictable, the past can't be changed, but life in the here and now is yours for the taking.

4. Minimize daydreaming. You know the feeling: you are sitting reading a book, studying a report or watching television, and ten minutes later you 'come to' with no idea what you've read or seen. Your thoughts have been a million miles away and those minutes are lost for good. We all solve problems by visualizing outcomes but that is very different from daydreaming. Problem solving this way is controlled thought leading to a decision, while daydreaming achieves nothing and disconnects us from the present. Whenever you find yourself daydreaming, bring your thoughts back to the here and now. If you spend just five minutes an hour daydreaming (which many of us can easily do) it adds up to 1 hour 20 minutes in every waking day, which mounts up to 9 hours 20 minutes every week. That's a whole day every week lost in daydreaming which could have been used for living.

5. Engage with others. We all need other people and they need us. Yet sadly, so often we don't fully engage with others until disaster hits and we desperately need their help. Phone a friend instead of surfing the Internet; chat with a flatmate or make the effort to ask a work colleague if they've had a nice holiday. Reach out and touch others with a kindly word, a smile or simply a friendly glance, whenever you can. Research has shown that each time we engage with another person 'feel-good' chemicals are released into the bloodstream. And engaging with others sets us firmly in the here and now.

Living in the present becomes easier the more we practise it.

Be aware, concentrate, don't dwell on the future or the past, minimize daydreaming, engage with others and you'll make the most of every day.

CHAPTER FIFTEEN

Express Your Feelings

Most of us accept that it is healthier to express our feelings rather than bottle them up. Research has shown that people who express their feelings lead happier and healthy lives; suffer fewer heart attacks, cancers and strokes. But expressing your feelings isn't always easy. While few of us would have a problem expressing positive feelings, for example, *I like your coat* or *That new hairstyle suits you*, or non-contentious feelings like *I'm very hungry* or *I'm too hot*, many of us become very anxious when we have to say something controversial: for example, *I don't want you texting your old boyfriend*, or *I really hate you using my nickname in public* or *I wish you wouldn't leave your nail clippings in the bath* or, to our boss, *I believe I am overdue for a pay rise.*

The reason many of us struggle to express our feelings in situations like these is fear: fear of the other person's reaction and that they will think less of us in the future. We all want to be liked and we don't want to be thought badly of. So we bottle up our negative feelings until we can't contain them any longer, and then they explode into anger and we say things we later regret. Either that or we continue to internalize our feelings, which results in gnawing frustration and low self-esteem, which seep out as irritability and all manner of physical and mental ailments.

However, the good news is that we can all learn how to express contentious feelings in a way that won't cause another person offence or to think less of us. In fact, expressing our feelings in an appropriate manner can cause others to think more highly of us and treat us with more respect. Here are a few simple guidelines for achieving this.

How to express negative feelings

1. **Identify and clarify your feelings.** This may seem obvious, but so often our feelings become confused, especially if we have been brooding on something for a while. Ask yourself what exactly you are feeling. Is it anger, jealousy, frustration, greed, guilt? Have you grounds for distrusting the woman you work with or is it that she was promoted before you? Be honest. If you are being eaten up by jealousy then admit it. Once you have identified the feeling then clarify the source. Ask yourself what exactly is causing the feeling – i.e. what or who is responsible for your anger/upset/anxiety. It may be a one-off remark by a usually good friend, or something more ongoing and insidious, such as

the attitude or behaviour of a work colleague towards you. It is important to identify and clarify what you are feeling so that you can deal with it appropriately.

2. Rate your feeling(s). On a scale of 1–10, how angry/hurt/ undervalued etc. do you feel? This is important because so often situations are misunderstood and escalate because the people involved are starting from different places, with different perceptions. This is especially true when men and women interact, as their perceptions can vary wildly. When the average man says he is hurt, he means he is badly hurt, big time, and it's going to take a lot of putting right. A woman may use the same phrase more lightly, in respect of a situation that a man might not even consider hurtful at all. Hurt, for example, might be the feeling that you are not being appreciated enough by your partner (rating 1–2); that you are the subject of ongoing malicious gossip (5–6); or that you are suffering from physical or mental abuse (9–10). By rating your feelings you will be able to choose the correct words to describe them to the other person, so reducing the chances of a misunderstanding occurring. A small hurt, with a low rating, could be expressed as *I was a bit put out that* ... while with a medium rating you might say *I was hurt that you* ... and a big hurt might merit *I feel very upset and angry by* ...

3. Ask yourself if you need to say how you feel. Once you have identified, clarified and rated your feelings, ask yourself if you need to express your feelings to someone else or if the matter is something you have to deal with. *Some things are better left unsaid* is a very true maxim. Some feelings are of our own making, for example jealousy, greed, guilt or unreturned love; no one else is to blame and we must deal with these feelings ourselves. There is nothing to be gained (and indeed much harm can be done) by expressing such feelings to another: *Andrew, I really resent you because you were promoted over me* or *Sally, I loathe you because you are happily married to my ex* are feelings that need to be kept to ourselves. Feelings of anger, rejection or being undervalued, on the other hand, are examples of feelings we may need to express to someone else. If Andrew is gloating and telling you every day that he was promoted over you, or if Sally makes smug comments that her marriage is working when yours did not, you would be justified in explaining to him or her that their comments are unnecessary, and ask them to stop making them. If another person says something that causes you pain then the chances are you are right to say how you feel.

4. Choose your moment. If you have decided you have a good reason to express how you feel, choose the right moment to do this. It should be at a time that suits both you and the person you are going to address, and it should be done in private – one to one, not in front of a large group. In an even tone, begin with the person's name, follow it with 'I' and prepare the person for what you are about to say.

'*Carol, I really need to talk to you. Is now a good time?*'

'Adam, I have something I need to discuss with you. Have you got a moment?'

'Jason, could I have a word, please, when you've finished with your mates?'

'Lisa, I need to talk to you when you've finished watching your television programme.'

An introduction like one of these, said in an even and calm tone, is non-confrontational and prepares the person, so that he or she knows you have something important to say. Once you have the correct moment and the person's attention, and the two of you are alone, you can begin.

5. Say it. Remembering the feeling you identified and rated, choose appropriate words, with the emphasis on 'I' not 'you'.

Aisha, I have a problem with the way you treat my mother …

Karl, I was hurt by the amount of time you spent with that girl at the party last night …

Mark, I am angry because …

Words like these are far better than something accusatory, such as *You're a self-centred pig who only thinks about himself!*
Continue with a brief explanation of why you are hurting, angry, etc.; then stop and wait for the person's response.

If there is silence, then wait some more. Remember that you have had days, weeks or even months to analyse and consider your feelings, while the other person is hearing them for the first time. He or she will be considering what you have said, thinking back to the situation, assessing their role, if they were guilty and what level of responsibility they should assume. Be patient.

6. Listen. When the other person starts to speak, listen carefully. Hear what they are saying, not what you think they will say, and don't interrupt or jump to conclusions. If the person apologizes – *I'm so sorry, I really didn't think I was causing you pain* – and the apology is sincere and unreserved, then accept it graciously (see below). If the person has apologized before for the same behaviour but not changed their ways (as can happen in a marriage or other close relationships), accept the apology, but point out that this has happened before and calmly discuss how the person will stop it from happening again.

7. Clarify. If the person has a problem remembering the situation that gave rise to your feelings, or believes he or she wasn't responsible for the way you feel and didn't do anything wrong, then you need to clarify. Maintaining a calm, even tone, and explain in more detail why you feel as you do.

David, I joined this firm because I wanted to advance my career as an accountant. Calling me 'sweetie-pie' and asking me to make the tea and look pretty when you have clients in isn't allowing me to do that. Indeed, I feel it is demeaning and undervalues my role as an equal member of this firm.

Then again wait and listen to what the person has to say.

8. Close. If you reach stalemate and the other person, despite you explaining how you feel and why, doesn't believe he or she has done anything wrong, then you need to close the conversation and give them time to reflect on what you've said – which they will. To continue the above example, you can say something like:

> *David, I'll leave you to think about what I've said. This matter is important to me; otherwise I wouldn't have mentioned it. I'm afraid we must agree to differ, but I would appreciate you not calling me 'sweetie-pie' in future.*

When you put it like this only the very unreasonable would take offence or not do as you ask.

9. Finish on a positive note and move on, whatever the outcome. You have expressed your feelings, handled the situation well (for which you can give yourself credit) and lifted the burden from your shoulders, so the other person is now aware of how you feel. End with something positive and appropriate. For example:

Thank you for your time. I feel this has given us a chance to air our views (when the person hasn't admitted responsibility and needs more time to reflect).

Thank you for being so understanding. I'm sure things will improve in the future (when the person has accepted a degree of responsibility).

Thank you. I knew you'd understand (when the person has admitted responsibility and apologized).

Now move on. You have expressed yourself and life is too short to hang on to negative feelings.

If you are responsible for someone else's negative feelings and they tell you how they feel, then show them the same respect and empathy you would expect to be shown. Listen to what the person has to say, consider your role in the feelings they describe and if you are to blame then say so and apologize:

I'm so sorry, I'd no idea I'd upset you.

I'm sorry, I'll try harder in the future.

It won't happen again.

As I've said before, none of us are perfect and recognizing when you are wrong and apologizing is a sign of a mature and rounded person. By doing so, you recognize that others need to express their feelings sometimes, just as you do to lead a happy and contented life.

CHAPTER SIXTEEN

Become Self-Reliant

My husband and my mother run my life. I always do as they say, even if it's not something I really want to do. I go along with their wishes to keep the peace, but I also know it lets me off the hook. If something goes wrong (like our holiday last year) I can't be blamed. I know I'm pathetic but how can I change?

I come from a traditional Asian family. My father was very strict (and domineering). He made all the decisions in my family and my mother never got a say. We all did what he wanted, all of the time. Now I'm married with a family of my own and I still leave all the decisions to my husband. It's causing a problem between us because he is a lot more liberal than my father and believes a husband and wife should decide things together.

I wish I could be more self-reliant. I'm twenty and live at university so you'd think I'd be independent, but I rely on my friends for everything. I don't do anything by myself. I knock for them before I go to lectures, shopping, the cafeteria and even the launderette! It's become a bit of a joke, although they are kind to me. I was the youngest of five children and every-thing was done for me at home. I never had to take the ini-tiative or do anything alone. I'm studying psychology so you'd think I'd know what to do to get over it, but it's not that easy when it's you!

I'm a thirty-one-year-old male and I rely on my partner for everything, and I mean everything. She even buys my under-wear! At work I have a responsible job and make decisions all the time, but at home I feel totally helpless. I expect my part-ner to assume all responsibility and run the house and under-standably she resents it. She says I'm putting on her. My father left us when I was a baby and my mother brought my brother and me up alone. She was always very strong and in charge. I guess I assumed my girlfriend would be the same when we lived together, which I know is unfair.

These extracts are from emails sent by readers who, for varying reasons, recognized they relied too heavily on others and needed to be more self-reliant, but were finding it difficult to change. We can probably all see traits of ourselves in these letters, with many of us feeling we should be more self-reliant. Self-reliance gives us confidence and a sense of accomplishment and fulfilment, making us happier and more contented. Being self-reliant says we are in charge of our lives, trust our own judgement, and are able to make rational and sensible decisions without relying heavily on others.

Self-reliance should begin to develop in childhood and then continue throughout our lives. A baby has no self-reliance but depends on its parents (or main care-giver) for everything – from being fed and kept clean to being safe and happy. Part of the parenting role is to develop a young child's self-reliance in line with the child's autonomy and independence. If children are encouraged to be self-reliant, then by the time they are young adults they will be making most of their own decisions and leading independent lives. Unfortunately many parents (often wanting to keep their children safe from harm) are over-protective. If children are denied access to the decision-making process by not being given responsibility, they never develop confidence in their own abilities and rely heavily on their parents. If left unchecked this can continue into adulthood, when they remain overly dependent on their parents, partner or close friend, resulting in frustration, under-achievement, low self-esteem and problems in relationships, as the writers above had found.

Adults vary in their level of self-reliance (for a number of reasons) but many of us can benefit from being more independent and having the confidence to say and do as we believe we should. I am not talking here about living life without the opinions, help, support and kindness of others – far from it. We all need others sometimes. Self-reliance is about being self-confident so that we are able to **take responsibility for our lives** and not be over-reliant or inappropriately dependent on others. It is also about knowing when to ask for help or seek advice from others as part of the decision-making process.

How to become more self-reliant

1. Always try before you ask for help. You are smarter than you think. If you are faced with a problem, try to work it out yourself, if necessary by researching in books or on the Internet. There is a vast amount of information now available on all subjects, so there is a good chance you will find the solution to your problem by typing the problem into a search engine or visiting the library. The sense of achievement you will gain by doing something you previously thought was impossible will be immense. Whether you are changing a light bulb or fuse, solving your child's maths problem, choosing clothes or building a house, before you decide you can't do it and ask someone else to do it (or worse, assume they will do it for you), try to do it yourself. I guarantee you will be surprised at just how much you can do. Each time you achieve something new your confidence will grow and eventually your mindset will be always to attempt something before asking for help. Look upon each achievement, no matter how small, as a stepping stone across the river to self-reliance.

2. If at first you don't succeed, try again. This is an old maxim but a wise one: keep trying to do what you have set out to do and the chances are that you will eventually succeed. Only ask for the opinion, advice or help of others when you are sure you can't do it.

3. Don't be afraid to take calculated risks. Life is one long learning process and if you never take a chance you will never achieve anything. Success will fuel your confidence and self-reliance and if you are unsuccessful you can learn from your experience or mistakes.

4. No one owes us. We are not entitled to anything, so don't assume others owe you. Once you are an adult no one – not even your parents, partner, loved ones or best friend – is automatically responsible for you. Don't put upon them. Take responsibility for your life; we have to work hard for what we gain.

5. Think and act positively. Have a philosophy and develop your goals and visions, as explained earlier in this book.

6. Congratulate yourself when you achieve something you didn't think you could. Whether it is removing a spider from the house (when you are arachnophobic), cooking a new dish or running a marathon, congratulate yourself. You have done something you didn't think was possible, all by yourself. Congratulate others who have achieved but don't expect them to congratulate you. You are not a child: you don't need others telling you how wonderful you are. You achieve for your own satisfaction and self-development. This is the path to self-reliance.

7. Help others. Share your knowledge and opinions with others when you are asked. It's a big compliment when someone values your opinion and experience enough to ask you for it. Not only will you be helping the person who has asked, but it will boost your confidence to be of assistance. Help the other person willingly but don't take over. Just as you benefited from attempting tasks yourself, so will others. It is crucial for our self-reliance to do things for ourselves.

CHAPTER SEVENTEEN

Develop Your Self

Just as we owe it to ourselves to make the best of life, so we owe it to ourselves to reach our personal best – through self-development. We are not all going to be champion chess, golf or tennis players, gain the Nobel Peace Prize, or become the Poet Laureate; indeed most of us won't even aspire to do so.

Self-development is not about competing with others but about **making the best of you for you.** It is about growing as a person, developing new skills and taking pride in your achievements. Self-development is a lifelong process where the only investment required from us is to be open to the new. We are never too old to learn, as is confirmed by the vast number of 'silver surfers' (elderly Internet users) who have taken up the challenge of learning the new technology, often rivalling their younger counterparts. You don't need a life coach for self-development: you have all the skills you need. No one is better qualified to work with you than you. You know yourself – your strengths and weaknesses.

The future is ours for the taking and self-development allows us to make the most of the future through learning and putting what we have learnt into practice. To make the most of ourselves we need to be not only **open to new ideas and experiences**, but also **willing to update and improve our existing skills.** Self-development is not the hard work it may at first sound: it is simply about being aware – aware of ourselves and of new opportunities, which present themselves daily. No, you don't have to read every night instead of watching television; nor do you have to sign up for activity holidays instead of relaxing on a beach. But you do have to wake up each morning ready to discover and accept what the world has to offer. Self-development is about enthusiasm and regaining a child's quest for knowledge.

An Individual Development Plan

Children at school often have an Individual Education Plan (IEP), which assesses their learning and sets targets for what they need to achieve. Similarly adults can have an Individual Development Plan (IDP). It's not as daft as it may seem; indeed many businesses especially in US already use IDPs for their employees. Your IDP does not have to be written down; you can just as easily hold it in your head, as long as you don't lose sight of it. Your IDP should contain where you are now in terms of your achievements (e.g. your skills, strengths and weaknesses) and where you want to be. It will contain a statement of intent.

A mother of teenage children might include in her IDP: *I have done a good job raising my family, but now there is time for me I'm going to research how I can get back into the job market.*

A newly retired person might include the statement: *I always worked hard at my job, and now I am going to do all those things I didn't have time for, beginning with learning to swim.*

A young business executive might include: *In order to advance my career I shall need to attend some weekend training courses but I also intend to make the most of the time I spend with my family on my weekends off.*

A student might say: *I am doing reasonably well in maths and science but in order to obtain the grades I need I will only go out with my mates once a week until after the exams.*

Self-development is not only about acknowledging where you are in your life and what you need to do to improve it but putting yourself in a position to do so. There is little to be gained by deciding you need to spend more time with your family if you are always at work; or that you want to develop your IT skills if you never go near a computer; or saying you want to learn horse-riding if you never take lessons; or deciding to learn a language if you don't join a programme to do so. In order to develop we need to put ourselves in the position of being able to learn and grow; otherwise our IDP is nothing more than a dream. We also need to be open to new, previously unconsidered possibilities. As long as we are still breathing we can change and grow.

A simple guide to self-development

1. Practise what you have learnt so far from this book. The techniques will allow you to develop a frame of mind from which self-development will follow naturally.

2. Be aware of what is going on in the world by watching the news each day on television or the Internet, reading a newspaper or listening to the radio. Being aware of what is going on in the world challenges us to think outside our comfort zone, puts our own lives in better perspective, and opens up possibilities for fuelling self-development.

3. Read whenever you have the chance – books, magazines, newspapers, journals; in bed at night, on the train, in the doctor's or dentist's waiting room. I've lost count of the number of really useful pieces of information I've picked up while sitting in my dentist's waiting room.

4. Open your eyes to what is around you, and practise seeing it through the eyes of a child. Children are like sponges in their thirst for knowledge: they soak it all up. All those apparently random questions young children bombard us with – *Why is the sky hollow? Why are my vegetables green? Why does the moon get smaller? Why do birds sing?* etc. – show their uninhibited thirst for knowledge. Ask yourself such questions as you did when you were a child and if you don't know the answer find out. It's a fascinating world out there but it is easy to forget just how fantastic, wondrous and unique it is. Recapture the wonder of childhood by asking why.

5. Visit places and travel, as far and wide as you can. Nothing opens the mind faster than being taken out of your bubble and into a different location or culture. Embrace it and learn all you can. If you can only manage an away day or a visit to a local place of interest, that is just as valuable.

> We have a very small museum in the next town to where I live; it has only two rooms but they are crammed to bursting with local artefacts and memorabilia. I have been taking children to this museum for twenty-five years and the display hasn't really changed much in that time, but I always come away having learnt something new, and so too do the children.

6. Try new hobbies and join organizations where you can share and discuss your interests. These clubs are often held locally in a library or church hall, nationally in city halls or in forums on the Internet. Listen to what others have to say and benefit from their wisdom, especially that of the elderly, who have so much knowledge and experience to offer.

7. Eliminate negative aspects of your personality: for example, being hypercritical, pessimistic or cynical, smoking, drinking to excess, etc. You and you alone hold the key to your self-development; you have the power to rid your life of unwanted baggage and all that is holding you back.

8. Have a role model. The writer Fay Weldon was mine for years. She had a young family but still found time to write, just as I was trying to do. Have a role model but not an idol: aspire to and learn from what that person has achieved, but don't idolize them or covet their achievements. I feel all warm inside when a reader emails me saying he or she admires my writing or the work I do with children, but I feel very uncomfortable when someone sets me on a pedestal and says: *You're fantastic. You're my idol, I could never do what you do.* Of course you could! I'm not a saint.

9. Regularly assess where you are and congratulate yourself on what you have achieved. Revise or confirm what you are aiming for.

10. Share your achievements. Self-development is not only about what you can achieve for your own benefit but also about sharing your achievements with others. We grow as people when we reach out to others and share. As one gentleman of eighty-six, living in a care home, wrote: *My son bought me a mobile phone last year and my grandson taught me to text. I showed it to the other residents and now most of us here has a mobile. We all text our family, friends and each other! The staff don't know.*

CHAPTER EIGHTEEN

It's OK to Be Sad (Sometimes)

By following the advice in this book you will greatly reduce the number of times you feel sad or unhappy, and will be on your way to lasting happiness and contentment. However, even the most happy and contented person feels sad or unhappy sometimes. It is part of life to experience 'highs' and 'lows'.

I make a distinction between sadness and unhappiness, and this is why. Sadness is usually acute and what we feel when we have lost someone or something very important to us, on the death of a loved one, divorce or the end of a friendship, for example; or when we are faced with a situation that's upsetting – for example, famine, an earthquake, a plane crash or a child being abused. Unhappiness tends to be ongoing, a state of mind that causes us feelings of frustration and discontent. Agonizing over the past, present or future causes us unhappiness, as does not being satisfied with what we have. Virtually all the 'lows' we all feel at some time fall into one of these two categories.

Sadness causes a more intense pain, resulting in us grieving, probably crying, and we gradually recover from it or learn to live with it. No one fully recovers from the death of a loved one but eventually, having gone through the grieving process, we learn to live with our loss and take comfort from the many happy memories we have of that person. Unhappiness, on the other hand, often brews and can fester from dissatisfaction – with a person, situation, or our lives in general. While it is perfectly natural to feel sadness and unhappiness sometimes, both need to be addressed, or else our health and well-being will suffer.

In order to address and deal with sadness or unhappiness we first need to identify the cause. Using the two categories I outlined above, here are the main causes for feeling sad or unhappy:

Sadness:

* death – of a loved one or pet
* divorce
* separation – from a loved one
* past or ongoing physical or mental abuse
* loss of a friendship
* loss of a job
* regret at a missed opportunity
* disappointed by an outcome
* ill health in ourselves or those we are close to.

Unhappiness:

* unaddressed anger
* unhappy marriage or bad family relationships
* not enough money
* lack of responsibility for your life
* dwelling on negative thoughts
* negative or anti-social behaviour
* no close friends or family
* lack of goals, visions or incentives
* poor body image and low self-esteem
* always seeing the worst in other people or outcomes
* stress
* jealousy
* frustration
* being overly dependent on others
* living in the past
* unable to express our feelings or true self
* drug or alcohol abuse
* fear of rejection or failure; fear of trying anything new
* turmoil in the country in which we live.

Sadness is more easily identified, as it tends to be incident led. You will be aware of what has happened in your life to make you feel sad, and know it is OK to be feeling sad, and possibly cry – that is appropriate and natural to do so. Those close to you will empathize with what you are going through, and give support and a shoulder to cry on. Not only will it be appropriate to be sad at this time but it will be important that you express your sadness as part of the eventual healing process.

Unhappiness, on the other hand, can be more difficult to identify, often because we don't want to acknowledge the cause (and therefore set about changing it), or because it has been part of our lives for so long we have accepted it as our base line. But the causes of unhappiness are identifiable, and as you go through the steps outlined in this book – letting go of anger, taking responsibility for your life and focusing on the positive, etc. – the cause of your unhappiness will become apparent. So you will be able to deal with it and eliminate or greatly reduce its effect. Of course, you are still going to feel unhappy sometimes, just as you will feel sad sometimes: that is normal. But having read this book you should be able to recognize the cause of your sadness or unhappiness and use the strategies you have learnt to deal with it.

It would be naïve of me, however, to say that once you make all the changes necessary to lead a happy and contented life you will never have a downturn or what we call an off day. This is when, for no good reason, you feel unhappy and at odds with the world. It may be you got out of bed with this heavy feeling or perhaps it descended on you as the day wore on. If this happens, acknowledge what you are feeling, assure yourself it is temporary and a normal part of life, and then give yourself a happiness boost to get you back on track.

A happiness boost

A happiness boost does exactly what it says on the packet. It is **an instant pick-me-up** that gives you an immediate lift back on to the path of happiness and contentment. It is not designed to offer long-term solutions to the areas in your life that are causing you unhappiness – the rest of this book does that. What the happiness boost does is to re-focus your mind and body (you will remember from earlier chapters that mind and body are so interconnected that they act as one, and therefore need to be treated together) so that you feel positive and happy. The happiness boost can be carried out anywhere and at any time.

1. Smile. When you smile, all those tiny facial muscles send messages to your brain telling it you are happy, and so you are. Smiling triggers happiness in the brain. Smile, in a mirror if there is one available; if not, just smile wherever you are. Feel the muscles in your face lift – your lips and mouth curve up; your cheeks rise; and your eyes open wide. Hold the smile for five seconds and repeat twice. Feel your spirits rise.

2. Relax. While you are smiling, consciously relax your neck, shoulders and arms. It doesn't have to be an obvious gesture if you are with other people, just a subtle loosening of these muscles. When you feel low you tense these muscles, even if you are slumped from lethargy or despondency. Relaxing them tells your brain you are no longer tense and, with the smile, makes you feel you are happy in your life.

3. Think positively. Our old friend positive thought again and for a happiness boost you need to focus on one thing you can look forward to. It doesn't have to be anything big: the thought of the nice meal you are going to cook when you get home can give you just as much of a happiness boost as looking forward to the holiday you are planning for the summer. Other happiness boost thoughts might be:

* leaving the office on time and going home to relax
* tucking up your little ones in bed for the night so that you can have some me time
* a game of tennis or round of golf
* phoning a friend and having a good chat
* making love
* buying a new outfit or even a bar of chocolate.

Think of something nice that you can look forward to and your spirits will rise from the anticipated pleasure. I know the promise of cake and coffee has seen me through many a gloomy meeting.

4. Jump. Star jump if you are somewhere where this is possible. As you jump into the air, spread your arms and legs as wide as you can. Your body will become buoyant and your mind will too. Six star jumps is all that is required to speed up your pulse, get the adrenaline going and kick-start your system into feeling good. Combined with steps 1, 2 and 3 it will give your happiness a big boost. If it's not possible to star jump (if you are in a meeting, for example), then stretch – your legs, arms and back – as much as is possible. You could drop your pen under the table and stretch to retrieve it; or if you are in a car, stretch as much as the space will safely allow. The movement of stretching will send blood rushing to your muscles and will kick-start your system, which, together with the smile, relaxing your muscles and a positive thought, will boost your happiness.

5. Enjoy the sun. UV rays which come from the sun have been given a bad press in the past, but recent research has shown that ten to fifteen minutes' sunlight a day on exposed skin (i.e. skin not covered by clothes or sun cream) not only boosts our immune system but instantly makes us feel better. This is because sunlight increases the serotonin levels in our bodies. Serotonin, you will remember, is the chemical that affects our mood and general mental health. It is nature's opium, a feel-good chemical, lack of which causes SAD (Seasonal Affective Disorder) in many of the population. Even in the middle of winter a blast of sunlight on our faces will help give us a happiness boost.

Use the happiness boost when you feel down and you will quickly shake off the gloom and feel the joy of life again.

Conclusion: I O It 2 Me

You are important. You have the right to be happy and contented. Life is a precious gift, full of opportunities, joy, love and experience. What you gain is only limited by the extent of your imagination. Of course life presents challenges, but they are character building and need not make you sad or unhappy, any more than you need to hold on to past anger. Having read this book you have the tools to deal with negative feelings, think positively and make the very best of your life.

This book could have been titled *I Owe It To Me*, for I firmly believe each of us owes it to ourselves to be happy and contented. Life is not a rehearsal and we get no second chances, so make the most of every day. I love the phrase 'I owe it to me'. It is my catchphrase and I have it stored in my phone. My friends know what I mean if I add *I O it 2 me* to a text: it tells them I am looking after myself, usually by taking 'me time', forgiving someone or getting rid of a negative thought.

If your life is not as good as it could be or you are hampered by negative thoughts and feelings, now is the time to change. The guidelines in this book are based on well-tried and tested practices that have been shown to work. Follow them and I am sure they will help. You owe it to yourself to be happy.

Remember

* Let go of anger.
* Take responsibility for your life.
* Think and act positively.
* Develop a positive philosophy.
* Have goals and a vision.
* Look after your body.
* Be body positive.
* Be optimistic and decisive.
* Listen to your intuition.
* Create a positive environment at home and at work.
* Reduce stress.
* Live in the present.
* Express your feelings.
* Become self-reliant.
* Develop your self.
* It is OK to feel sad sometimes.

And lastly key *I O it 2 me* into your phone as a little reminder of the **importance of you.**